The Heart of the Breath

'I struggle to think of a more capable and committed professional in the world of voice care. Alison has an extraordinary skill in rehabilitating complex vocal injury, through a thorough understanding of detailed anatomy and physiology, both at a laryngeal and holistic level. It has been a privilege to share patients with her.' - Ed Blake (Laryngeal and Vocal Physiotherapist)

'I am so grateful for Alison's contribution to my progress and development as a vocalist, in particular the rehabilitation of my voice post-surgery. It is a pleasure to have been able to learn so much from her about keeping the voice safe and healthy. I recommend this book to anyone who wants to further their knowledge about the voice, its recovery and retaining vocal health.'
- Nathan Sykes (Singer/Songwriter)

'Watching Alison work, you know that you are in the presence of a complete professional. She has a wealth of technical knowledge, along with the ability to precisely discern the most suitable exercises for her rehabilitation clients. Aware that she is dealing with artists and an art form, Alison is passionate about helping singers restore their voices and is acutely sensitive about the negative impact that voice problems can incur. Her book radiates warmth and clarity, reflecting her holistic approach and including artful illustrations that make anatomy user friendly.'
- Clare Costa (Singing Teacher and Voice Therapist)

Vocal Health and Rehabilitation: Clinical Pathways and Practical Applications Series

Series Editor: Alison Mary Sutton

This series of books represents a comprehensive resource for singers, singing teachers and all those seeking to understand more about the injured voice.

Practical and easy to read, each book in the series incorporates clearly structured practice routines, with helpful tips for their application backed up by instructive audio and video clips. Collectively they present a portfolio of detailed vocal rehabilitation case studies which reflect the Author's extensive experience in this field. Illuminating illustrations by artist, Meg Pike, in close collaboration with the Author, reinforce a concise and digestible approach to each topic area.

Alison Mary Sutton's insightful fusion of voice with yoga and psychology will help readers to build up a picture of why voices can run into trouble and how remedial work is undertaken. She highlights in each book the importance of re-establishing the magic and joy of singing, as well as mapping the hard methodology. Aiming to make the understanding of vocal rehabilitative techniques more readily accessible, these titles will be essential reading for those who want to engage with this topic at a deeper level.

The Heart of the Breath

Alison Mary Sutton
Illustrations by Meg Pike

A volume in the Vocal Health and Rehabilitation:
Clinical Pathways and Practical Applications Series

compton
PUBLISHING

This edition first published 2023 © 2023 by Compton Publishing.

Editorial offices: 35 East Street, Braunton, EX33 2EA, UK
Web: www.comptonpublishing.co.uk

The right of the author to be identified as the author of this work has been asserted in accordance with the UK Copyright, Designs and Patents Act 1988.

All rights reserved. No part of this publication may be reproduced, stored in a retrieval system, or transmitted, in any form or by any means, electronic, mechanical, photocopying, recording or otherwise, except as permitted by the UK Copyright, Designs and Patents Act 1988, without the prior permission of the publisher.

Trademarks: Designations used by companies to distinguish their products are often claimed as trademarks. Any brand names and product names used in this book are trade names, service marks, trademarks or registered trademarks of their respective owners. The publisher is not associated with any product or vendor mentioned in this book.

Disclaimer: This book is designed to provide helpful information on the subject discussed. This book is not meant to be used, nor should it be used, to diagnose or treat any medical condition. For diagnosis or treatment of any medical condition, consult your own physician or registered allied health professional. The publisher and author are not responsible for any specific medical condition that may require medical supervision and are not liable for any damages or negative consequences to any person reading or following the information in this book. References are provided for informational purposes only and do not constitute endorsement of any product, website, or other source.

Permissions: Where necessary, the publisher and author(s) have made every attempt to contact copyright owners and clear permissions for copyrighted materials. In the event that this has not been possible, the publisher invites the copyright owner to contact them so that the necessary acknowledgments can be made.

All text and images © Alison Mary Sutton unless otherwise indicated

ISBN 978-1-909082-67-0

A catalogue record for this book is available from the British Library.

Cover design and typeset: Matt Oakley, Mojo Design Studio. www.mojostudio.co.uk

Dedication

In memory of my mother,
Alice Stevenson Sutton (1919–2021)
one of many victims of COVID-19

Contents

Dedication	iii
Acknowledgements	v
Foreword by Neil Mackie, CBE	vii
Foreword by Sara Gourlay	viii
Introduction	1
1. The heart of the breath	12
2. Case study: Muscle tension dysphonia in a contemporary commercial music (CCM) singer	55
References	124
Index	126
About the Author	128

Acknowledgements

I would like to offer my thanks to all the people who assisted and supported me in the development of this book, including Anne Pain, Clare Costa, Carol Tayler, and Phil Sadler, for his assistance with the finer points of YouTube. Sincere gratitude for the tireless encouragement from the late Jeffery Babb, formerly Head of Music at Wintringham School, Grimsby, where it all began. Thanks, too, to Sara Gourlay and Professor Neil Mackie for their kind words in their Forewords to this book.

I owe special thanks to Michael Hardingham, retired Consultant ENT Surgeon, for enabling me to start on the rehabilitation pathway as an observer in the voice clinic at Cheltenham General Hospital, and subsequently Consultant ENT Surgeon, David Michael Thomas and Principal Lead Speech and Language Therapist, Jane Haxworth. They have generously shared their medical expertise on voice related issues, providing a rich resource of knowledge for which I am hugely grateful.

Sincere thanks are also extended to Ed Blake for his expert and much-appreciated comment on anatomical detail.

It would be impossible to name all the vocal rehabilitation clients who have contributed to the content of this book and from whom I have learnt so much. Grateful thanks to them for sharing their vocal struggles and vulnerabilities, which provided the invaluable insight and understanding that inspired the writing of this book.

The editorial expertise and support from Noel McPherson of Compton Publishing has consistently steered my understanding of the relationship between writer and publisher.

Heartfelt thanks to my illustrator, Meg Pike, for her masterful drawings, endless patience, enthusiasm and attention to detail. Countless hours have been spent together in planning and discussion at Jaffe and Neale Bookshop and Cafe, Chipping Norton, to whom I also offer thanks. In addition, I wish to remember the help and support of Lisa Hopton and Danny Blyth for clarification of illustrative anatomical detail.

Finally, I offer immense gratitude to my husband, Richard, who has constantly supported me in the process of writing, without which this book would never have been written.

Foreword

Alison Mary Sutton has gained a wide and enviable reputation as a practitioner of vocal rehabilitation. Her excellent book is a welcome addition for pedagogues, medics, singers and students alike.

As former Head of Vocal Studies at the Royal College of Music in London, I know Alison's outstanding work from personal experience. I recommend without reservation her hugely informative study, complemented by distinctive academic research.

Professor Neil Mackie, CBE.

Foreword

I first met Alison in 2015 when I engaged her as a speaker on my Canto Lecture Series. She was booked to give a lecture and workshop on singing rehabilitation, which proved to be a popular and highly regarded event.

In my capacity as a Speech and Language Therapist (SALT) and singer, I subsequently visited the voice clinic at Cheltenham General Hospital, where Alison is on the team as Singing Rehabilitation Coach following many years of clinical observation. It was clear that the multi-disciplinary approach with the ENT consultant and SALT was beneficial for the patients, with Alison's opinion being sought where appropriate. Professional boundaries were respected throughout, and I came away in the knowledge that she was on top of her brief and took the interest of singers' vocal issues very seriously.

Alison has a profound and thorough understanding of the anatomy and physiology of the singing voice alongside a clear awareness of the problems and distress that can arise when things go wrong. This is supported by many years of experience as a singer and singing teacher. She is methodical, meticulous, and painstaking in her approach to rehabilitation, ensuring that her clients have the best chance of success and leave her studio feeling empowered and better informed about their vocal wellbeing. Above all she is compassionate and caring and truly understands the tragedy of vocal problems for singers, an essential quality in this demanding role.

This book is a wonderful testament to her work, and there is something for everyone here. She has written a comprehensive and illuminating case study, in which she has been generous and open in sharing her expertise. This is nothing more than I would expect from someone who continues to put singers in trouble first.

Sara Gourlay
Singer, Speech & Language Therapist
and Vocal Rehabilitation Therapist (Retired)

Introduction
Finding my way

The Heart of the Breath is the first in a series of practical books: Vocal Health and Rehabilitation: Clinical Pathways and Practical Applications.

It features extensive coverage of the principles of breathing that I have formulated with rehabilitation clients over a long period, coupled with a detailed client case study that demonstrates, practically, how these principles have been successfully applied. The complete series will contain further case studies and illustrated chapters, including rehabilitation and yoga technique, as well as vocal psychology and performance.

Vocal science and pedagogy have advanced beyond all recognition in recent years and continue to be widely researched and documented. I am grateful to have been a part of this era, having attended many courses and heard inspiring presentations by the people who have been in its vanguard. My writing is a practical contribution of how I have put this knowledge into practice, combined with many years' experience of singing, teaching singing and vocal rehabilitation work in studio and in a voice clinic.

I will demonstrate the connection between these different aspects, and how they have enabled me to help rehabilitation clients to rediscover their voices.

The contents are by no means the definitive version, but rather my interpretation of all that I have learnt. I am fully aware of the complex vocal science that lies behind my instruction. Whilst it constantly informs my work, it cannot be applied to all the techniques referred to in this book which, nevertheless, have proved effective over time.

By using a case study and suggesting practical tips, I am able to highlight the degree of detail required to achieve, where possible, a positive outcome for rehabilitation clients. My approach is systematic, which is reinforced by all sessions being recorded so that clients can work with them afterwards in their own time. The instruction given in the case study is chosen to suit the client's individual needs, including the basics of singing technique. The hope is that this book may encourage a preventative approach that can be incorporated into the singing teaching studio, helping singing teachers to recognise what could be happening if a pupil is giving cause for concern, perhaps because of an uncomfortable vocal sensation or ongoing symptom. Having this awareness is crucial when trying to decide if it is appropriate to advise a pupil to seek a referral from a general practitioner (GP) to an ear, nose and throat specialist (ENT) for further investigation.

Having been involved with a hospital voice clinic for many years, the knowledge that I have gained has helped me to develop both my rehabilitation work and singing teaching in equal measure. Over time, they have complemented each other in an increasingly positive way, backed up by my long-standing practice of yoga and breathing. What I have discovered, largely due to this long association with yoga, is that the breath is everything! It underpins all forms of voice work and, if utilized optimally, can enhance vocal longevity as well as the various aspects of the performance 'package' – that is: phrasing, vocal tone/range, dynamics and interpretation. It has become the keystone of my rehabilitation work, as the majority of clients have developed problems due to habitual under- or overpowering the voice, which can then easily become exacerbated by continuing to sing when unwell – for example, with a viral cold, upper respiratory tract infection or laryngitis.

There have been numerous instances in my teaching career that have clearly shown the need for a personal approach to voice training. No two students are the same, and each will inevitably interpret instruction differently. The voice is ever changing, and its development or recovery must be tailored to fit each person individually. Equally necessary has been the realisation that the teaching process is not just about giving instruction, but about enabling the transformation of a voice and the blossoming of a singer's emotional wellbeing through appropriate vocal development. As the voice is an integral and unique part of a singer's identity, I see it as essential to invite a sense of teamwork as I work alongside clients, helping them to explore and discover their own vocal potential and fulfilment of personal expression.

I started singing at the age of six, when I joined the school choir. We were taking part in a local festival, and I can still remember the excitement and apprehension of performing to an audience. These two feelings imply psychological conflict, and yet in a performing situation they can be surprisingly compatible. It all depends upon them being in balance with each other. As I grew older, I began to explore solo repertoire, which intensified my love of singing. I recall the joy of performing in my teenage years, when singing felt instinctive and allowed me full rein to express myself. At that point, the excitement of performing far outweighed the apprehension, with nerves never threatening to overwhelm me. I was always fully engaged in telling the story and living in the text, moment by moment, unaware that my active imagination was allowing me to access vocal colour naturally. I heard the term 'vocal colour' mentioned many times when I was at music college, but by then I was grappling with the complexities of singing technique and my imaginative skills began to take a back seat. Consequently, vocal colour as an interpretative tool often eluded me as a professional singer. I finally understood its significance many years later, when I heard accompanist Malcolm Martineau define it during a masterclass: 'Vocal colour is a response to the play of feeling in the music and text. It is a reflection of the psychology of the moment.' By that time, my technique was secure enough to have regained the freedom of self-expression, and I was able to put this maxim into practice. Prior to this point, my singing tended to be rather hit and miss, and not many performances passed without experiencing crippling nerves and the uncertainty of whether apprehension would outweigh the excitement. As every singer knows, this is a very uncomfortable and potentially destructive feeling.

At age 18, I secured a place at the Guildhall School of Music and Drama, London. I was very reassured to be accepted, it having previously been suggested by a respected local singing teacher that I would not make it as a professional singer. This remark overshadowed my college years, as it gave me the feeling that I had had my wings clipped before I had even got started! However, I pursued a successful career in opera, oratorio and recital, singing at major London concert halls and with opera companies including Kent Opera, London Opera Factory and Opera de Lyon, travelling widely in the UK and Europe.

I consider myself to be most fortunate in the way that my professional life evolved over the years, embracing more activities than I could ever have imagined. Most of them ran alongside my singing career and collectively led eventually to my involvement with singing rehabilitation. A part-time job as a primary school music teacher allowed me to hone my teaching skills, and I briefly enjoyed running a music appreciation class for homeless men in a rehabilitation centre for the Inner London Education Authority (ILEA), as part of its adult education programme. A complete contrast was my examining and adjudicating work, which fulfilled my enthusiasm for encouraging singers of all ages to explore their vocal potential. I helped to train a choir by instructing small groups of its members on basic singing technique, which led to my starting a singing teaching practice. As time went by, I gradually became more specialised, giving masterclasses, running my own singing course and acting as external examiner for undergraduate and postgraduate level recitals at Birmingham Conservatoire. I continue to keep active as a singer, believing it necessary to maintain the muscular coordination and physical sensations of singing in order to successfully convey them to others. Being able to create musical vibrations across a wide harmonic range on every sung note produces an intense feeling of wellbeing, which

I am inspired to pass on to clients. As long as there is no diagnosed vocal pathology that prevents access to the precise muscular movements required, they can be encouraged to have the same experience via the same techniques. Not only does this engender confidence it also allows the voice freedom to find its own way to optimal vocal function.

As I got older and my singing career began to slow down, I attended several Estill Voice Training System (EVTS) courses and became very interested in vocal anatomy and physiology. At this point I was most fortunate to be given permission to observe in the voice clinic at my local hospital. This was the beginning of a long learning journey that gradually led to many ENT patient referrals and finally culminated in my becoming the singing rehabilitation coach in the clinic. From the outset, I started to appreciate the link between vocal science and the art of singing, realising that having a clear perspective of both made it possible to see the way in which each enhanced the other. I also began to find it easier to understand specific vocal challenges that some of my pupils were experiencing, and it was with a sense of relief that I felt more informed in seeking ways to help them.

And then disaster struck on a personal level – or so I thought at the time! Following a diagnosis of breast cancer, subsequent surgery and chemotherapy, I experienced a bad depression. Over a long period, and without a real understanding of what was happening, I had neglected to address a personal bereavement whilst at the same time continuing to work and support others. The final trigger was the chemotherapy, to which my body reacted very badly. According to medical advice, full recovery could take up to three years and I certainly think that this was true in my case. Those desolate years felt like crossing a wasteland, but gradually the joy of life began to reawaken in me.

Once recovered, all my senses seemed heightened, and I could once more fully engage with life. Recognising my immense good fortune, I now wanted to make the most of it. I had always been interested in psychology and I decided at this point to develop it further, with a view to gaining a better understanding of how I might prevent reoccurrence of such a frightening experience. This study with a personal mentor has proved invaluable; I have not only gained greater personal insight from his learned and compassionate approach but have also been taught how to address the inevitable psychological distress of singers who come for vocal rehabilitation. This comes up time and time again with clients. Guidance by my mentor, a professional psychotherapist, has enabled me to recognise and take appropriate approaches to the management of clients who may have suffered some sort of abuse, including one case directly related to singing. To help rebuild someone's self-confidence, as well as their voice, is immensely rewarding. I have learned a huge amount about stress management since my recovery and have found that personal experience has added an extra dimension when offering advice to clients. This includes the development of an awareness that encompasses compassion towards oneself as well as towards others. In addition, I have learned about respecting professional boundaries, giving me a clear understanding of where one can and can't venture with vulnerable clients. This goes hand in hand with being able to evaluate the appropriate information to convey. I am led by my clients and have found that any emotional aspects directly relating to singing and the voice tend to surface in the second or third session. To be entrusted with personal confidences is a huge privilege. If this responsibility can be handled with skill and sensitivity, it can hopefully result in the unlocking and giving back to another human being the precious tools of vocal and artistic fulfilment.

In writing these books, I want to look at ways in which singers can maintain the heart and health of their singing for as long as possible. Most importantly, my aim in working with any aspect of the voice is to encourage and regain the joy of singing: When successfully harnessed to the imagination and the intent to communicate, it enables our fundamental need for self-expression to emerge, whether in performance or everyday life.

Alison Mary Sutton
October 2022

Publisher's Note

Throughout the book there are links to audio-visual files. These files can be heard or viewed on YouTube at https://tinyurl.com/nhheph5k

The heart of the breath

'How singers think they use the respiratory apparatus in singing and how they actually use it are often very different things'

This quote, from Thomas Hixon's *Respiratory Function in Singing* (2006), highlights breathing as being one of the most contentious issues in the singing world.

Hixon went on to posit that optimal respiratory function *'accelerates and enhances the development of performing skill, minimises performance fatigue, increases the dynamic range of the voice and maximises the economy of performance'*.

In the Introduction, I identified breathing as having become the keystone of my rehabilitation work. My experience with most of my clients is that they have developed vocal problems due to some form of breath mismanagement, leading them to either over- or underpower the voice. Singers can run into difficulties if there is a perceived need to have a 'big voice', especially in the operatic field. Choral singers can experience problems as a result of having restrained their voices, often unwittingly, in order to blend with those around them. Most of my chorister clients share common issues of vocal strain and fatigue, often due to low breath pressure, weak onset and tongue root tension (TRT). In all cases, symptoms have manifested as a result of differing degrees of prolonged vocal restraint. Insufficient understanding of respiratory function can lead to unhelpful muscular compensatory patterns becoming entrenched, whereas having clear understanding has, as Hixon states, *'the potential to extend performance life through the prevention of misuse and abuse of the singing apparatus, and the prevention of certain injuries that might interrupt performance life or threaten its continuation'*.

Over the years, I have observed a common challenge with rehabilitation clients regarding a particular aspect of breathing, which spans all vocal genres and frequently turns out to be the primary cause of vocal tension and distressing symptoms. In addressing this aspect, I have given emphasis to practical work, with reference to theoretical points of breathing and anatomy that aim to substantiate it within a clear framework. It concerns my gradual recognition that one of the most crucial aspects of maintaining vocal health and longevity is the subtle balance between inhalation and exhalation. This balance can easily become out of sync in singers, especially when quick inhalation is needed between successive and demanding phrases, for example in high impact opera singing and belting. I began to realise that the key to achieving it relies on learning how to disassociate from the deeply ingrained 'fight and flight' survival response, especially on inhalation. It is the sympathetic nervous system (SNS) which triggers the body into this mode of operation, in order to mobilise resources of energy to face challenges that are linked to anxiety or fear, such as a predator... or a performance! This tends to induce gasping of air and lifting of the shoulders, often followed by rapid deflation of the lungs and potential loss of vocal control. When this happens, the refinement of diaphragmatic action necessary for healthy singing can become compromised, with potential detrimental effect on the vocal folds (see 'Regulating diaphragmatic action in singing' p.48). Engagement with the parasympathetic nervous system

(PNS) can help to override these tendencies. It engenders a more relaxed response which lowers blood pressure and slows the heart rate, calming anxiety and allowing blood to flow more easily into tight and potentially over-reactive muscles. Yoga masters discovered centuries ago that abdominal breathing is directly connected with the PNS and has a generally calming effect. Once a gentle and rhythmic breathing pattern is established, the PNS engages naturally and takes over from the SNS 'fight and flight' response (see Balloons analogy, p.28). This helps to redress exhale/inhale imbalance, allowing greater vocal control. It also helps to reduce the 'freeze' element of the 'fight and flight' response that can so readily manifest in pre-performance nerves, or even make an unwelcome arrival when standing on the platform.

It is generally much easier for a singer to activate the vocal folds for sound production than it is to control the air intake between phrases. Healthy voicing depends on the exhale/inhale balance being consistently maintained through differing phrase lengths and at all dynamic levels. Achieving this balance relies on mastering appropriate airflow through the vocal folds on every phrase, which was highlighted to me at a British Voice Association course, 'How the Breath Inspires'. Presented by Ed Blake[1], a pioneer of physiotherapy treatments for singers with vast experience in the management of performance-related injuries, it included a screened demonstration of abdominal ultrasound imaging. I signed up to take part, and duly succumbed to having the imaging probe placed on my lower abdomen before sirening to different sounds. The outcome was highly informative, as it demonstrated in visual terms the order in which the different abdominal muscles engage when phonating. To illuminate, sirening on 'NG', 'ZZ' and 'VV' showed the following under ultrasound imaging:

> 'NG' siren – mainly transverse abdominal muscle (TA) engagement on ascent, followed by the internal oblique muscles (IO) towards the top of the range as the pitch and breath pressure rose. IO engagement continued to be maintained on descent.
>
> 'ZZ' siren – TA engagement on initial ascent, with IO engaging sooner than 'NG' and at a deeper level, due to the breath pressure being higher and more resistant

---

[1] www.physioedmedical.co.uk (accessed May 2021)

to the airflow than the 'NG' siren. As the pitch rose, the imaging resembled a layered river of rippling muscular movement, with the TA engagement remaining consistent.

'VV' siren – further resistance to the airflow reflected an even greater depth of IO engagement, which maintained consistency and flow/fluidity throughout the siren.

It was noted that there was little engagement of the external oblique muscles (EO) during the sirens. Being the outermost abdominal muscular layer, there is less involvement in the control of breath pressure and airflow.

This exercise was very significant, as it clarified the crucial role that sequential muscular engagement plays in maintaining healthy vocal function and preventing potential vocal problems, for example, dysphonia (see Case Study). Achieving this in practice enables accuracy of subglottic pressure and pitch control through precise regulation of diaphragmatic action, which is discussed later in the chapter.

The abdominal muscles form the abdominal wall, giving the body a stable base from which to move (known as core stability). This allows general dexterity of other muscles and the limbs. Along with quadratus lumborum and rectus abdominis, they consist of three flat layers (see Figures 1 and 2). They are, from the innermost to the outermost, transverse abdominal, internal and external obliques. The transverse abdominal moves horizontally forward, the internal obliques upwards and forwards and the external obliques downwards and forwards. Extending between the vertebral column, the lower ribs, the iliac crest and pubis of the hip, their fibres merge towards the midline and surround the rectus abdominis in a sheath before joining up on the opposite side at the linea alba. Always in control of active exhalation, abdominal muscular strength is gained by the interlocking of the muscular fibres. Figures 1 and 2 are schematic rather than medical illustrations, designed to demonstrate the principle of how the fibres interlock and the muscles function on exhalation and inhalation.

The transverse abdominal muscle (TA), also known as transversus abdominis, is the deepest layer, wrapping horizontally from the back to the front of the body, acting as a muscular corset. It consists of upper, middle and lower fibres, with the middle fibres being the most dense. Connecting the last six inferior ribs and the iliac crest to the linea alba, there is a transition point between the diaphragm and the TA, where the fibres oppose each other at right angles (see Figure 5). This transition occurs where the inner surfaces of the TA rib cartilages intersect with six corresponding diaphragmatic connections. The TA is the main driver for exhalation and singing, with an engagement of between 60-70% for opera and belting. It doesn't connect directly to the spine, but the fascial connective tissue surrounding it goes all the way around to the outside of the lumbar spine. With its function being to compress the abdomen, any exhalation where there is heightened resistance to the airflow should automatically bring the TA into play, for example when playing a wind instrument or blowing up a balloon. This also applies to singing, "*...as the TA is the fundamental muscular contributor to maintaining stable subglottic pressure levels. However, singers with high movement backgrounds, who may be predisposed to using their obliques in a phasic manner, may not automatically use the TA as the primary abdominal muscle in generating subglottic pressure. Conversely, when used in a static, low-level activation, it can be argued that the obliques provide an anchoring and scaffolding facility that allows for improved TA control*" (Blake, Pers. Comm., 2020).

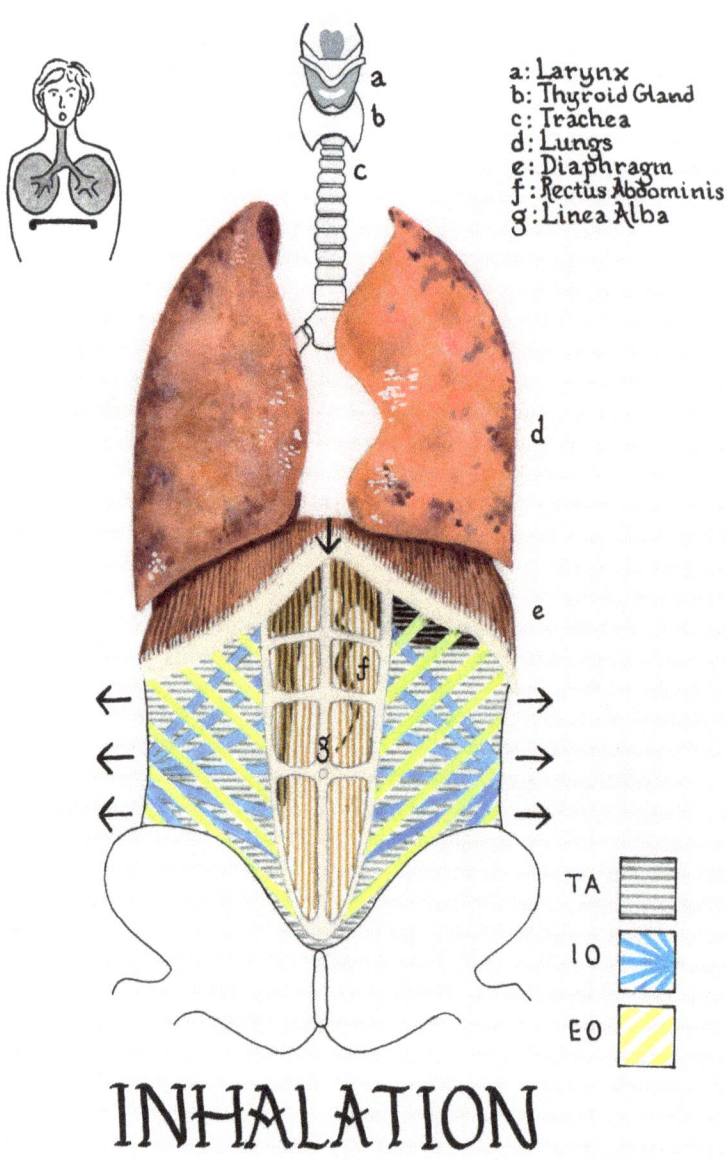

Figure 1. Layering of the abdominal muscles (Inhalation)

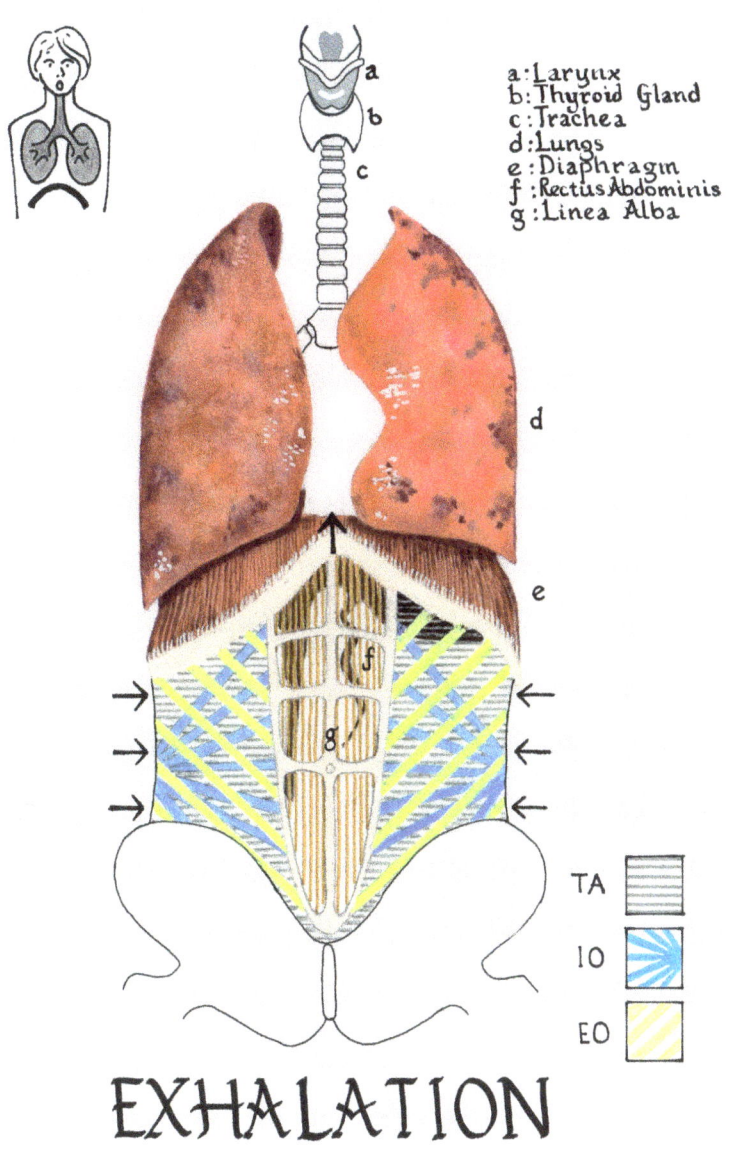

Figure 2. Layering of the abdominal muscles (Exhalation)

The internal obliques (IO) lie above the TA on the mid/lower half of the thorax. Key to generating airflow, they are core muscles connecting the iliac crest to the intercostal cartilages of ribs 8–12. Acting as an antagonist to the diaphragm, they help to reduce the volume of the chest cavity during exhalation. When the IO contract, they compress the organs of the abdomen, pushing them up into the diaphragm, whose resulting ascent into the chest cavity causes a reduction in the volume of the air-filled lungs, producing an exhalation.

The external obliques (EO) are the outermost abdominal muscles, lying above the IO and to the sides of the rectus abdominis. They extend from the lower half of the ribs around and down to the iliac crest, covering the sides of the abdominal area. As well as supporting the flexion and rotation of the trunk and spine, they allow compression of the abdominal cavity and assist in exhalation. They are essential for postural stability, especially in dancers.

The rectus abdominis (RA) is a pair of long, flat muscles that extend vertically in the front of the abdominal wall, covering the entire length of the abdomen adjacent to the umbilicus. Running between the pubic bone and the sternum, it acts as a centre post and is important for maintaining postural alignment. Each muscle consists of four muscular bodies, connected by narrow bands of tendon. When well defined and tensed, it gives a bumpy appearance, resulting in its nickname 'six-pack'. RA helps in keeping the internal organs intact, and in creating intra-abdominal pressure, such as when exercising or lifting heavy weights.

In respiration, the RA plays a crucial role when forcefully exhaling, such as during exercise and in conditions where exhalation is difficult, for example, emphysema. However, as far as singing is concerned, it is often referred to as 'no-man's land'. This is because over-engagement of the 'six-pack' can compromise an optimally supported airflow, which relies on flexibility in the navel area. It is critical that the upper RA should feel soft and flexible when singing, in order that the lower RA can engage and disengage appropriately.

In his presentation, Ed Blake stressed that muscle tension dysphonia is more likely to occur if the ratio (workload) between the transverse abdominal (TA) and internal obliques (IO) is similar, that is, 1:1. This is because consistently high-level IO activity in conjunction with TA activity creates constantly high subglottic pressure, causing a potential imbalance of delicate laryngeal strap muscle activity and length. *"Receptors present just below the glottis are very sensitive to these pressure levels, and sustained high subglottic pressure is believed to trigger a compensatory muscular response in the sternocleidomastoid (SCM) to limit the detrimental effect of this sustained high pressure on the vocal folds. It is essentially a self-protective response, but should this environment exist for any prolonged period, then secondary changes in the length and activity of the supra and infra hyoid musculature can be observed"* (Blake, Pers. Comm., 2020). It was apparent in the ultrasound imaging demonstration that the IO engage as both pitch and breath pressure rise, resulting in greater depth of function due to the increase in airflow resistance. For this reason, the IO are referred to as the 'turbo' muscles. It is imperative that they are not active all the time, otherwise the load on the vocal folds is too great. Too much engagement can lead to the voice being over-supported, with subsequent abdominal tension and rigidity. Equally vital is the need to disengage and 'turn off' the IO on inhalation, otherwise the transition of airflow between exhale and inhale can become compromised and inhibit its free movement through an appropriately positioned larynx. *"If the obliques remain constantly engaged, achieving abdominal wall relaxation as part of the passive recoil on inspiration is very difficult, and may lead to chronic use of proximal breathing patterns and associated muscular tension in the cervical and upper thoracic spines. Abdominal relaxation is also critical in achieving appropriate TA engagement for the subsequent outbreath"* (Blake, Pers. Comm., 2020).

Singing teaching inevitably puts a lot of focus on abdominal breathing but, as Ed Blake underlines, preserving good muscular balance is essential. Over engagement can restrict free movement of the ribcage and adversely affect airflow, potentially compromising optimum vocal fold vibration. Being the deepest layer, and firing milliseconds before the other muscles, it is crucial that the TA leads at the start of a phrase, as was seen in the ultrasound imaging demonstration. This was highlighted by one of my 'belter' rock and pop clients, who I had rehabilitated following successful surgical removal of a vocal polyp. He had been habitually over-engaging his IO when belting, and not disengaging them sufficiently between phrases. As a result, he was experiencing an uncomfortable sensation of weakness as he transitioned from the middle to upper register, often being tempted to play safe and revert to his belting 'set up'. This was denying him the ability to produce a softer sound on the transition notes, when the lyrics frequently demanded a less intense emotion. He found it helpful to see visuals of the abdominal muscles during inhalation and exhalation (Figures 1 and 2) and could appreciate the relevance and importance of isolating the TA (grey) from the IO (blue), on which he had been relying too heavily. Using the breathing exercises below, he gradually achieved the necessary precision and balance of the TA/IO relationship. This led to an outcome of healthier singing and more convincing performances, as he was able to draw on greater vocal colour and dynamic control across his full vocal range.

The breathing exercises in this chapter are aimed at helping to create the conditions that encourage both TA control and appropriate sequential abdominal engagement. Muscular stamina can then be built up gradually, so as to be able to sustain long phrases without collapse of the chest wall and subsequent 'fight and flight' inhale. Whilst working on them, it is preferable to take more frequent breaths when singing until breath pressure is fully regulated. Once accomplished, the abdominal muscles should be able to soften and retract between every phrase (they possess an elastic property which allows them to do this at differing speeds), enabling optimum contact of the vocal folds throughout every phrase. Being an internal instrument that can neither be seen nor touched, it is challenging for singers to trust that there can be a positive effect on vocal tone if they concentrate on core muscular sensation rather than internal listening when creating efficient exhale/inhale balance. This is particularly relevant when having to take quick breaths in a short space of time. The question is, how can this balance be ultimately relied upon as the foundation of vocal longevity and optimal performance?

I have been a Vinyasa yoga practitioner for many years, which has consistently informed my understanding of the power of the breath. The fundamental emphasis of this tradition is that the breath is the medium for all movement. Through continual focus on the combination of breath and movement in yoga postures, I gradually became aware of the vital connection between the breath and the body. Each posture is undertaken slowly and is carefully synchronized with smooth and focused breathing. I also began to realise that the principle of Ujjayi (throat breathing) matched perfectly with that required for singing and healthy vocal function. It is a relaxing exercise which I introduce to all clients, as it lays the foundation of the more strenuous breath work that follows. As confusion can often arise with clients when questioned about breathing, I precede the exercise by using a balloon analogy to demonstrate the way that the lungs react to two different breathing patterns. It effectively clarifies the necessity to disassociate from the deeply ingrained 'fight and flight' inhale response:

> Balloon A is inflated and released. It whirls around noisily and empties rapidly as the air pressure falls. This action corresponds to the rapid deflation of the lungs on exhalation, as there is no resistance to the airflow. It is usually followed by a 'gaspy' inhalation, creating an uncomfortable and shallow breathing pattern.
> This comparison reflects the sympathetic nervous system (SNS), where inhalation tends to be short and

quick, often accompanied by rising of the shoulders.

Balloon B is inflated, and the neck stretched to make a valve, which slows down the rate of escaping air. This action corresponds to the slower deflation of the lungs on exhalation, as there is resistance to the airflow due to having created a valve.
This comparison reflects the parasympathetic nervous system (PNS), where inhalation is calmer and deeper. It should be accompanied by abdominal muscular release, with no lifting of the shoulders.

The breathing exercises introduce airflow resistance to the inhalation as well as exhalation, in order to help override the instinctive gasping of air, as demonstrated in Balloon A. To maintain healthy and deeper breathing function, it is vital that singers and wind players learn to adopt the Balloon B system. Although the principle is the same for both, wind players need to generate lower airflow and higher breath pressure than singers, who need to generate moderate airflow and moderate breath pressure for optimal voicing. Time and patience are essential when establishing the Balloon B system, as it is very different from everyday breathing. It also plays a significant part in the respiratory 'braking' process (see 'Regulating diaphragmatic action in singing' p.48.

When doing the exercises, most clients initially experience a sense of panic when applying airflow resistance to inhalation, feeling that they can't access enough air or that they are running out of breath. This can be due to an instinctive drive to empty the lungs before breathing in (they do, in fact, always contain some residual air). The introduction of airflow resistance to the inhale helps to override this instinct and encourage a 'topping up' of the remaining air in the lungs. A crucial aspect of diaphragmatic function helps to enable this action (see 'How does the diaphragm fit into all this?' p.42).

Throat valve breathing exercise (Ujjayi)

The primary function of this exercise is to establish an equal length of inhalation and exhalation at the site of the glottis, that is, between the vocal folds. It is a low resistance airflow technique, which encourages a natural lengthening of the breath. By partial closing of the glottis and narrowing of the proximity of the vocal folds, the friction of the air passing through them creates a valve, resulting in a soft hissing sound that resembles waves breaking gently on the shore. Establishing a rhythmic breathing pattern begins to isolate and strengthen the transverse abdominal muscle (consisting of the innermost muscular fibres of the core of the body), as it engages and disengages on exhale/inhale respectively. The lips remain gently closed in the exercise, allowing the breath to flow naturally in and out of the nostrils. It is best practised lying on the back, when the higher position of the diaphragm and chest wall enables the wider range of movement necessary for deep breathing.

In this exercise, the drag on the airflow on inhalation acts as a temporary crutch, encouraging a weakening of the body's instinctive trigger of pulling or gasping in the air, as described in Balloon A. It encourages and allows the respiratory system to adopt and strengthen the abdominal inhalation response, as described in Balloon B. Initially, it can take a few minutes for the breath to settle into a relaxed rhythm, which can be more challenging when feeling stressed or having just engaged in active sport. When repeated on a little and often basis, this exercise can gradually calm and settle the nervous system, creating a long-term muscle memory that ultimately allows abdominal release to be reproduced without conscious thought. Concentrated effort can then be applied to greater effect elsewhere.

Instructions for throat valve breathing exercise

 Audio clip 1 – throat valve breathing exercise
NOTE: AV files can be heard or viewed on https://tinyurl.com/nhheph5k

1. Lying on the back, place the thumbs on the navel and the fingers on the lower abdomen. Breathe in and out naturally for a few seconds.

2. With the mouth closed, begin to make the sound 'HAH' in the throat on both exhalation and inhalation. This creates a valve effect, and should result in a soft hiss, along with a sensation of the narrowing of the proximity of the vocal folds. It may be noticeably more challenging to maintain the 'HAH' and hissing sound on inhalation. If so, try to match the exhalation length to an inhalation length that can be comfortably managed.

3. Continuing the 'HAH' sound, observe the natural rise and fall of the abdomen/navel as the breath becomes more even and rhythmic. (This movement is more readily perceived by women in the lower abdomen, who generally find release in this area easier than men, who are more likely to feel it in the navel area). As the breath settles, try to establish an equal exhale/inhale ratio of approximately four seconds, counting inwardly. Once established, follow this up with 6–12 perfectly balanced breaths for full benefit to be achieved.

4. Keeping the valve effect of the 'HAH' on exhalation, relinquish it on inhalation by opening the mouth and *waiting* for the air to enter the lungs without conscious involvement. Having already become accustomed to the automatic rise of the abdomen on inhale when using the resistant 'HAH', allow the body to continue to make the same movement without it.

Finger valve breathing exercise

This exercise works on the same principle as the throat valve breathing but uses a moderate resistance airflow technique that is more appropriate for singing. It is best attempted when the throat valve breathing exercise has been comfortably assimilated, as it activates the deeper internal oblique muscles that require greater physical stamina. For this reason, maximum benefit is gained by practising it in a standing position, as it is easier to access the movement of this deeper muscular pattern when erect. Being vocal athletes, singers need to increase core strength on a gradual basis, recognising appropriate abdominal engagement/disengagement without causing muscular strain or unwanted tension. As with the throat valve breathing exercise, importance is given to equalising the length of both exhalation and inhalation at a constant and moderate pressure, which acts as the basis for ultimate safe singing in terms of volume, vocal range and pitch.

The forefingers are used like a reed to create a valve and moderate resistance to the airflow (see Figures 3a and 3b). The friction of the air passing through them produces a more robust hissing sound than the throat valve breathing exercise, as there is higher breath pressure and greater glottal closure. Similar to the principle of Semi Occluded Vocal Tract (SOVT) exercises[2], where the airflow is semi-closed off, this is an exercise which is used in a rehabilitative context to focus solely on muscular abdominal precision, as it is an imbalance of this function that frequently presents with clients. It should be accompanied by a sense of muscular 'gathering' of vitality in the abdominal core which, through repetition and recognition, gradually restores confidence and trust in breathing function. If the airflow through the fingers is too forceful or too weak, the resulting sensations in the core are noticeably less vital, producing either tension and discomfort or barely being felt at all. The principle of using the forefingers in this way correlates to the reed of a wind instrument. In the case of a wind player, optimal airflow through the reed is achieved by creating an embouchure, where the lips, facial muscles, tongue and teeth are engaged to seal the area around the mouthpiece. This serves to prevent air from escaping whilst simultaneously supporting the reed, allowing it to vibrate but at the same time employing pressurised airflow to constrict it appropriately and prevent too much or too little vibration. Using the forefingers to emulate a reed activates the appropriate balance of breath pressure below and above the vocal folds. This balance is called inertance, an acoustic concept that allows them to operate most efficiently, enabling the balance between breath pressure

---

[2] https://www.voicescienceworks.org/straw-phonation.html (Accessed March 2023)

from below and acoustic back pressure from above the vocal folds to be maintained. Acoustic back pressure occurs when the different energy boosts of the vocal tract align with harmonics such that energy returns to the vocal folds (Titze, 2001, pp.520–23; Svec, et al, 2021, pp.4–5). Without optimal inertance vibration, the load on the vocal folds can become too great and potentially cause damage.

Care has to be taken with this exercise, as it can induce a temporary feeling of dizziness, as in blowing up a balloon. This occurs as a result of the Valsalva manoeuvre, where moderately forceful exhalation through a closed glottis can elicit cardiovascular responses. Due to a faster pulse rate, it increases pressure in the chest, lowers heart rate and reflexively causes blood vessels to constrict.

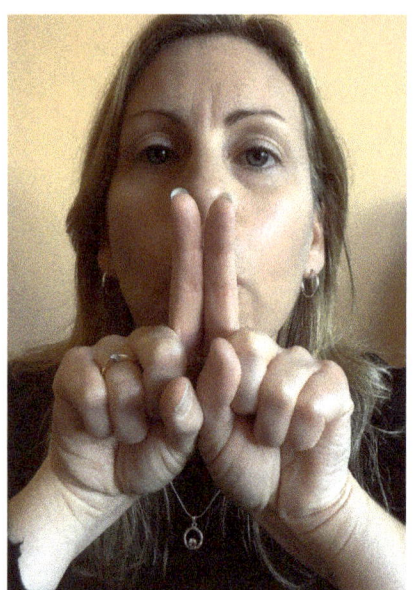 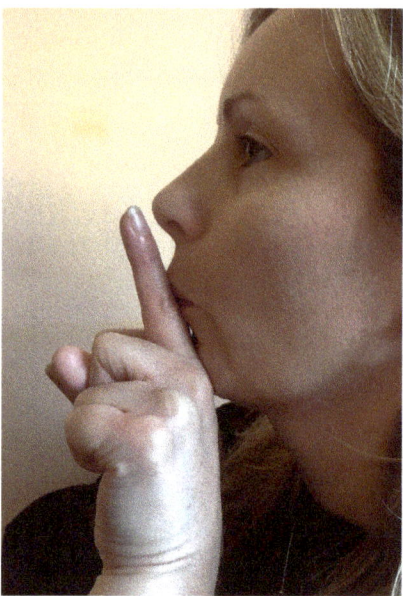

Figures 3a and 3b. Position for finger valve breathing exercise.

Instructions for finger valve breathing exercise

 Audio clip 2– finger valve breathing exercise

1. Standing up, place the forefingers in a vertical position and bring them together so that they are gently touching (see Figures 3a and 3b). Like a wind player preparing the embouchure prior to playing, purse the lips and press them against the knuckles, creating a valve. Blow air through the knuckles for approximately four seconds. This should produce a moderately loud hissing sound, which needs to be even and consistent. Repeat several times until comfortable, at the same time gradually becoming aware of an accompanying sensation of muscular 'gathering' in the abdominal core. If this sensation is not felt, it will be due to the breath pressure through the fingers being either too low (resulting in weak and breathy airflow), or too high (resulting in over engagement of the core and possible tension in the neck and shoulders). Withdraw the fingers in between each exhalation, allowing the core muscles to release and the air to flow gently in through the mouth.

2. Keeping the fingers in a vertical position, blow through them for four seconds and then inhale through them for the same length of time (as if sucking in through a partially blocked straw). The hissing sound should be identical for both, with disengagement of the core on inhale. This can feel quite strenuous, in which case stop and rest. Gradually build to an equal exhale/inhale ratio of approximately four seconds, counting inwardly. Repeat on a daily basis, but for FOUR BREATHS ONLY.

3. When 1 and 2 have been comfortably assimilated, and there is awareness of an even 'piston like' movement in the navel/abdominal area, start to remove the fingers for each alternate inhalation. Keeping an approximate four second exhale/inhale ratio, maintain the valve effect by using the fingers on exhalation, but relinquish it on inhalation and *wait* for the air to enter the lungs without conscious involvement. Repeat four times.

4. On the two inhalations without the fingers, open the mouth slightly to 'receive' the incoming air, waiting as long as necessary for the body to trigger automatic abdominal release. This may initially take longer to happen, due to a slower response of the deeper muscle fibres. The goal is to achieve an identical sensation of abdominal release on inhale, both with and without the fingers. Repeat these four breaths daily.

Video clip 1 - demonstration of 1 and 2 above

Matching the length of exhale and inhale allows sufficient time for adoption of the Balloon B system. Inhalation can then start to be shortened without jeopardising exhalation by creating unwanted muscular tension. I use a numerical table as a guide to progressive inhale shortening, in which the valve principle is applied to encourage assimilation of a natural sense of flexible, muscular vigour (see Figure 4). In this way, the transition is made to becoming a true vocal athlete, as demonstrated in the extract from Bizet's *'The Pearlfishers'* (https://www.youtube.com/watch?v=y3xyp54bZqs - Video clip 2).

Audio clip 3 – finger valve exercise working with the numerical table

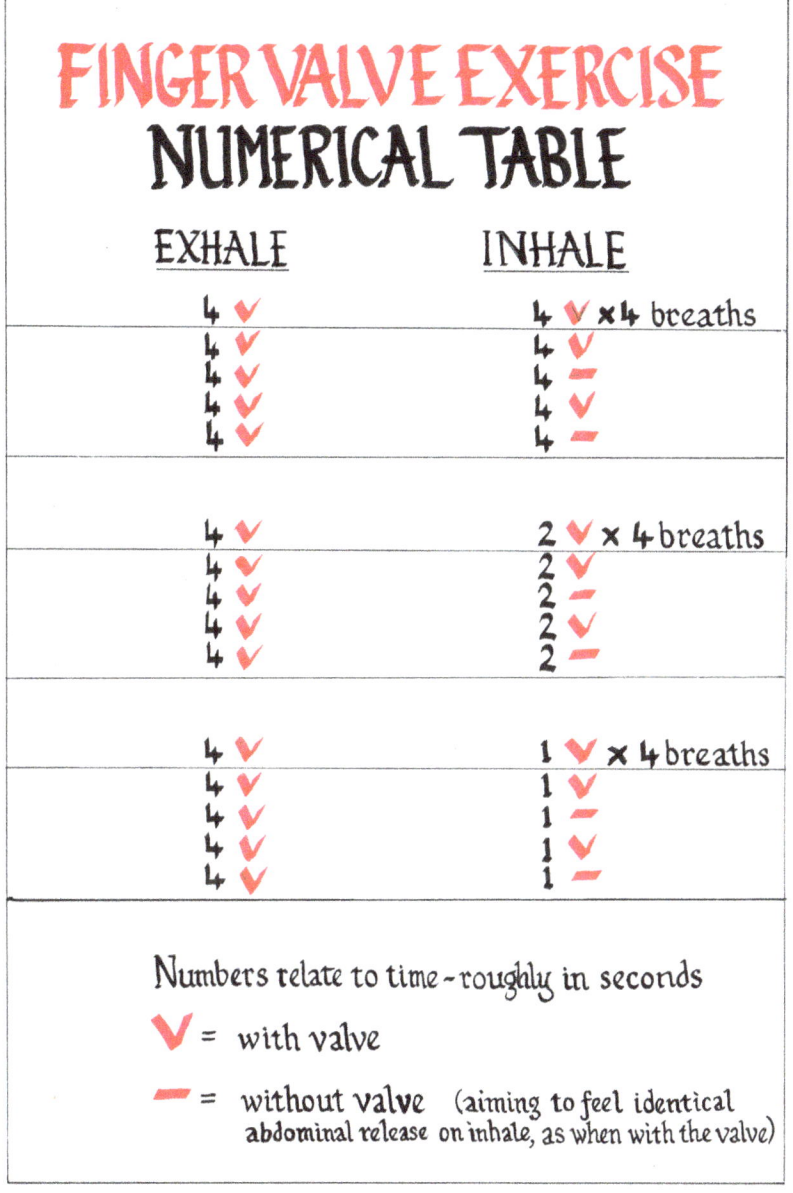

Figure 4. The finger valve exercise numerical table

How does the diaphragm fit in to all this?

Although inextricably linked to breathing, I tend to avoid mentioning the diaphragm to clients until they have a clear understanding of the principle on which the breathing exercises are based. This is due to diaphragmatic function being a controversial aspect of singing, which can arouse considerable confusion. Over the years I have been fortunate and grateful to have heard experts such as Ed Blake, Meribeth Dayme, Janice Chapman and Ron Morris give presentations on this topic, which helped clarify the crucial role that the diaphragm plays in singing. Although vital in achieving optimal vocal function, the diaphragm is not completely under our voluntary control. As a result, conscious movement of it is limited, which can present a significant challenge for singers.

Writing about the diaphragm in his book, *Discover Your Voice*, Oren Brown states that it is the most important muscle for breathing. He goes on to say that *'to gain a proper understanding of how the diaphragm functions, it is important to know that its motion is influenced by posture'* (1996, p.18). Having evolved from a four-legged species, he refers to the need for human beings to work on good posture and a flexible ribcage, adding that *'four-legged animals have no problem in keeping their ribs expanded. Babies go through a stage of crawling before they walk'*. It is worth noting that crawling babies, like four-legged animals, travel forwards with their eyes aligned along the same horizontal plane as the spine. Once upright, this alignment changes, in that the eyes remain directed along the horizontal plane, but the vertical spine is now at right angles to the direction in which the body is travelling. Over time, the potential stress that this can put on the spine is what therapies like the Alexander Technique seek to address. Oren Brown cites Mabel Todd, one of the pioneers in the mind/body wellness connection, and her book *The Thinking Body*, in which she states that as an infant develops, *'active movements and the resultant deeper breathing bring about the coordinated action of the entire spine. This process is greatly aided by spells of crying and screaming, since the diaphragm and the lower lumbar and pelvic muscles are so closely associated'* (1937, pp.94, 251).

The diaphragm is a muscular partition that separates the thoracic chest cavity from the abdominal cavity. It acts like *'a 'double-sided tape' between the two, adhering to the thoracic cavity via the pericardium (which surrounds the heart) and the pleura (which surround the lungs), and the abdominal cavity via the peritoneum (which envelops most of the abdominal viscera). Consequently, the diaphragm unites the two cavities, with displacement in one of them having repercussions on the other'*. This connection between the two cavities means *'that their mechanical properties interact, which is one key to the generation of the voice, explaining how subglottal pressure can be created by displacement of the abdomen'* (Germain, et al., 2016). Being attached to the pleura, which in turn is loosely attached to the rib cage, the diaphragm and ribs cannot make any movement without affecting the lungs and changing their shape. Along with the muscles of inspiration, the diaphragm plays a key role in controlling airflow in and out of the lungs.

Sitting up inside the rib cage, the diaphragm is a thin dome-shaped muscle which acts like an elastic stocking cap over the abdominal organs (viscera). It consists of vertical muscle fibres, which at one end converge at the top of the dome and attach to the central tendon, a thin layer of interlaced fibres which join at various angles to form bundles, which give the diaphragm its strength. They are responsible for lowering the diaphragm on **inhalation**. The other end of the vertical muscle fibres attach to the inner surfaces of the cartilages

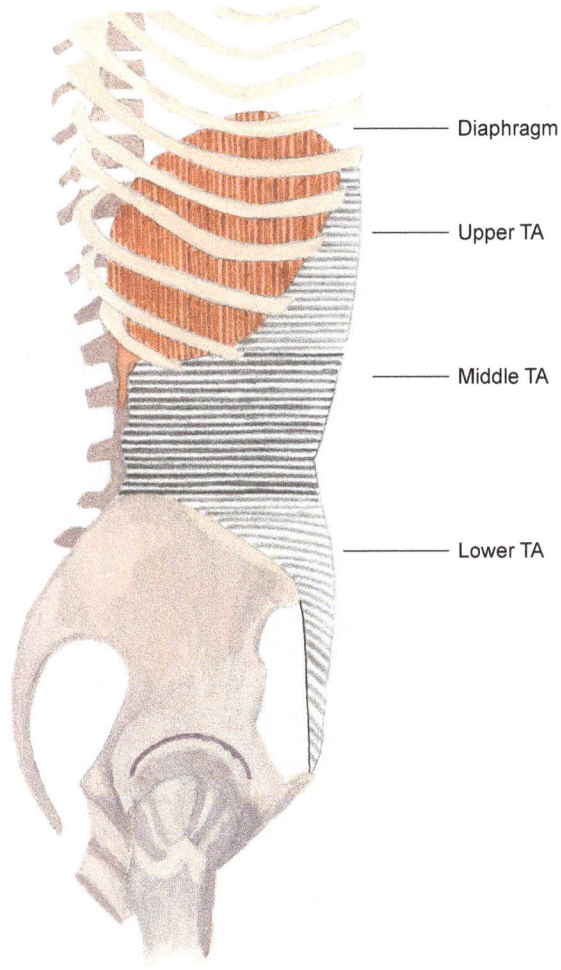

Figure 5. Diaphragmatic attachments to the ribs and transverse abdominal muscle (TA). Image after Keleher (http://sensational-yoga-poses.com).

of the lower six ribs, from the front edges around to the spine. At the front edges, they intersect with the horizontal transverse abdominal (TA) muscle fibres (see Figure 5). *"This interdigitation allows for a complete and connected structure, with the diaphragm positioned as the apex and the TA as the sides of a balloon. Contraction of the TA can then control apical elevation, allowing for consistent subglottic pressure levels"* (Blake, Pers. Comm., 2020). The TA muscle fibres lengthen as the diaphragm descends on inhalation, allowing the lower ribs to widen and expand. At the same time the upper ribs increase front to back expansion of the body.

The shortening of the diaphragm fibres results in compression of the viscera, displacing the abdominal contents. At the same time, the descending diaphragm pulls the lower wall of the chest cavity down, creating a vacuum effect that draws air into the lungs. This is due to the negative pressure created as the chest cavity increases in volume and expands. Air from outside automatically enters the lungs to balance the pressure [3].

In everyday breathing, **exhalation** is a passive action, promoted largely by the recoil of soft tissues with no conscious expiratory muscle activity. The resulting fall in air pressure allows the diaphragm to relax and rise. Along with serratus

---

[3] Boyles Law www.teachmephysiology.com/respiratory-system/ventilation/mechanics-of-breathing (Accessed March 2023)

posterior, the abdominal muscles are the main drivers for active exhalation. Contraction of the internal obliques and TA compress the organs of the abdomen, pushing them up into the diaphragm. Its resulting ascent into the chest cavity causes air to be expelled from the lungs as they reduce in volume and become smaller. The external obliques also assist in exhalation, as they allow compression of the abdominal cavity.

Although a possible link between muscular tension and emotional stress is not fully understood, scientific studies have shown that muscle tension may play a role in anxiety disorder[4]. If this is the case, the diaphragm is potentially one of many muscles whose function could be adversely affected by tension as a result of emotional stress. This would inevitably have a negative impact on breathing, as was demonstrated by one of my clients, who had been experiencing a lot of stress and presented with a very shallow inhalation. What was interesting was her positive response to the finger valve breathing exercise. She clearly had sufficient stamina to master it successfully and was able to access a deeper breathing pattern when using the fingers to provide airflow resistance. I attributed this anomaly to the fact that she walked everywhere and was physically fit. As she continued to work on the exercise, her normal inhalation began to deepen and become stronger. At the same time, she found that the rhythmic pattern of the throat valve breathing exercise had a calming effect on her anxiety.

---

[4] https://www.sciencedirect.com/science/article/abs/pii/S088761850800090X (Accessed March 2023)

Regulating diaphragmatic action in singing

We breathe thousands of times a day, mostly without conscious thought. This is one of the reasons why problems can arise when singers 'learn' about breathing, as they have to navigate the potentially hazardous route of achieving a more conscious response, which involves modifying the action of the diaphragm. In everyday breathing, the rise of the diaphragm on exhalation is a passive action, when the air pressure is continually falling. When singing, however, the regulation of subglottic pressure relies on higher air pressure being maintained below the vocal folds, which would indicate that the rapid fall of air pressure on a passive exhale is inappropriate. Instead, there needs to be a way of delaying the upward ascent of the diaphragm on exhale, in order for a singer to be able to regulate subglottic pressure and airflow. This would allow a sustained vocal line to be maintained and avoid compromise to vocal health. An unsteady airflow can result in an unsteady larynx...and the dreaded wobble! *'The interdigitation between the TA and diaphragm is important here, as it provides some voluntary control of diaphragm elevation in what historically, is a proven proprioceptor-free structure, which acts in isolation without voluntary control'* (Blake, Pers. Comm., 2020). Facilitating this crucial upward braking effect is also aided by exerting specific control of the diaphragm's downward movement on inhale (see Balloon B system p.29). *'Increased lung volume and capacity is accessed by using the external intercostal muscles in conjunction with a relaxation of the abdominal wall, allowing for an outward movement of the lower thorax'* (Blake, Pers. Comm., 2020). This is the key factor in the breathing exercises, as they generate the appropriate muscular flexibility to maintain the diaphragm's flattened inhale position for longer, reinforcing its action as a releasing brake on exhale (Morris, 2014). With sufficient muscular stamina, it is also possible to briefly maintain the diaphragm's flattened position as the exhale starts, giving a precious opportunity to extend the breath for the following phrase.

There is another factor to mastering this aspect of diaphragmatic control, which demonstrates the link between technique and interpretation. The moment of silence between phrases, when time momentarily stands still, can be magical! If the inhale can be taken in such a way that allows the diaphragm to be maintained in its flattened position for longer, it provides a singer with a bridge between phrases, across which the subtle changes of textual thought can be transmitted. Such moments enable an audience to anticipate what is coming next, both musically and textually, potentially intensifying the performance experience.

Posture

In the previous section, Oren Brown is quoted as saying that *'to gain a proper understanding of how the diaphragm functions, it is important to know that its motion is influenced by posture'*. This reinforces the importance of optimal postural alignment when regulating diaphragmatic action during singing. Achieving the highly refined inhale/exhale muscular balance is very much dependent on this, with good postural alignment often being referred to as the 'noble posture' of singing. It also stabilizes skeletal structure and provides the body with a firm base from which to move. Except at moments when high impact vocal power is needed, stiffening the spine in vocal work should be avoided, as it can cause postural tension instead of allowing flexibility between the sacrum and occiput at the base and top of the spine. The following considerations are essential to efficient breathing and voice production.

- Optimum posture allows flexibility in the spine, ribcage and intercostal muscles, along with mobility in the thoracic area. This helps diaphragmatic function by creating the space for greater lung capacity.

One of the reasons why voice teachers give much attention to posture and breathing is because of the need for an efficient supply of air in singing.

- The lungs are elastic filled sacs, and postural alignment is very relevant when it comes to their vital capacity and air volume. Normal, quiet breathing is referred to as tidal volume, when only a small amount of air is being used, and there is always some left in the lungs. The amount of air left in the lungs after a forced exhalation, such as sighing, is referred to as residual volume. The vital capacity of the lungs uses the full range of volume over and above residual volume and is essential for effective abdominal breathing. It allows greater lung expansion, resulting in greater air pressure being available on exhale. Access to the vital capacity of the lungs requires good postural alignment, which is why it is so important for singing.

- Optimum posture assists the muscles of inhalation and exhalation to achieve maximum diaphragmatic function, so as to enable efficient movement when breaths have to be taken quickly in a short space of time.

- The core posture of the body is stabilised by the diaphragm, in which it plays a secondary role to that of its primary one of breathing. When singing, the adoption of a deeper breathing pattern facilitates greater oxygen absorption. During this process, the diaphragm more consistently adopts a lower position within the core of the body. This is especially evident during deep breathing, where its lower position increases intra-abdominal pressure (IAP) and serves to stabilise the lumbar spine. *'The results of the study provide evidence that the diaphragm and TA muscles continuously contribute to respiration and postural control. The mechanical consequence of contraction of the diaphragm and TA is an opposing action on the rib cage and abdomen but a shared function for pressurization of the abdominal cavity. Postural function is relevant to changes in respiratory muscle function with exercise'* (Hodges and Gandevia, 2000). In singers, therefore, when the position of the diaphragm is lower through deep breathing, it assists in strengthening the core, highlighting the importance of muscular stamina and athletic endeavour.

Earlier, I mentioned that when rehabilitating clients 'there is a common challenge that spans all vocal genres regarding a particular aspect of breathing'. In my emphasis on practical work, I have addressed the nature of this challenge, making theoretical points on breathing and anatomy where appropriate. Those involved in vocal training know that there isn't a 'one size fits all' approach to singing, and I have been mindful of the need to adapt the breathing exercises from client to client and voice to voice. Common to the human body, however, is the breathing apparatus. It is a miraculous system of muscular levers and pulleys which, when balanced in perfect harmony, functions like a delicate and well-oiled clock mechanism. Over many years of developing my rehabilitation work, it has been evident time and again that clients need to find this point of balance in order to restore vocal confidence and wellbeing.

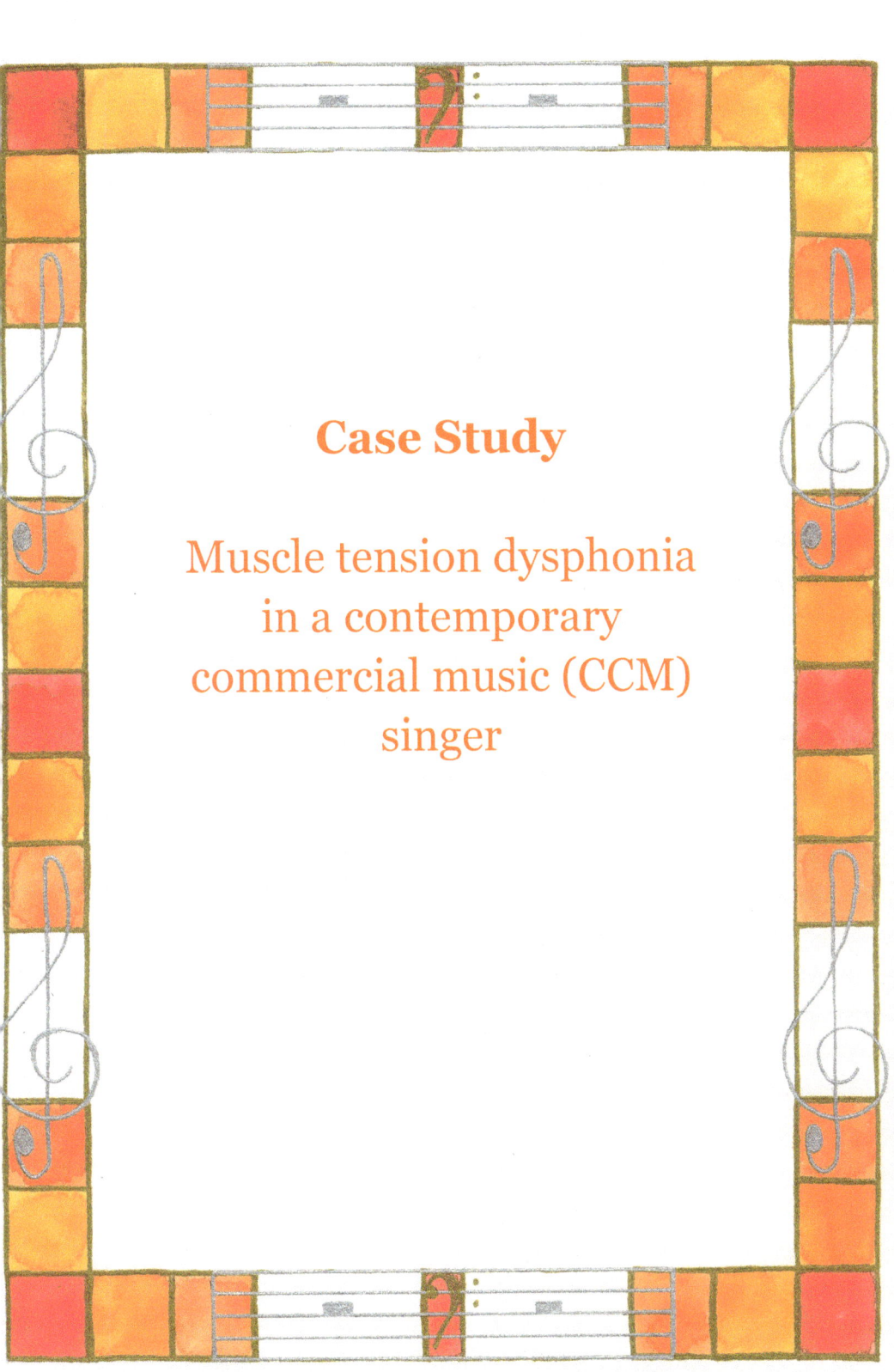

Case Study

Muscle tension dysphonia in a contemporary commercial music (CCM) singer

Diagnosis

Ethan, aged 27, was a rock singer who had been performing in bands for over ten years. He had developed a problem with his vocal range, experiencing a feeling of strangulation when trying to sing higher notes that previously had been easily accessible. His breath was noticeably running out quicker and he had a feeling of vocal fatigue after singing for only a short period. This was causing him concern and distress, combined with a fear of losing his voice altogether. ENT investigation revealed laryngeal tension (muscle tension dysphonia), but there was no specific vocal fold pathology. He was advised to see a singing rehabilitation specialist.

Ethan was dedicated and determined, with a committed approach to his rehabilitation. He fully understood the necessity to be systematic in his practice, working gently at muscular co-ordination and realignment in order to achieve full and lasting recovery of vocal function.

Rehabilitation

Ethan's contemporary commercial music (CCM) vocal style included high impact belting and the extreme effect of vocal distortion[5]. Prior to diagnosis, his voice had started to falter in these areas, which both involved his upper range. These vocal qualities necessitate having to draw on maximum output of vocal energy for short periods, with little room for error, as the vocal mechanism is balanced on a knife edge. Although some singers have a natural aptitude for belting, the voice is still totally dependent on expert handling to deliver the spine-tingling intensity of such a loud and vibrant sound. Failure to achieve this can result in vocal collapse just at the point where a singer is needing to convey the most intense emotions in the lyrics.

Over the period of ten years that Ethan had been singing, his vocal mechanism had been put under increasing strain. He had managed on raw talent and vocal intuition alone, but without the necessary tools to handle his voice efficiently, distressing symptoms had begun to appear. This had led to the laryngeal musculature becoming tight and tense, resulting in a diagnosis of muscle tension dysphonia (MTD).

---

[5] https://completevocal.institute/distortion/ (Accessed March 2023)

What does Muscle Tension Dysphonia look like?

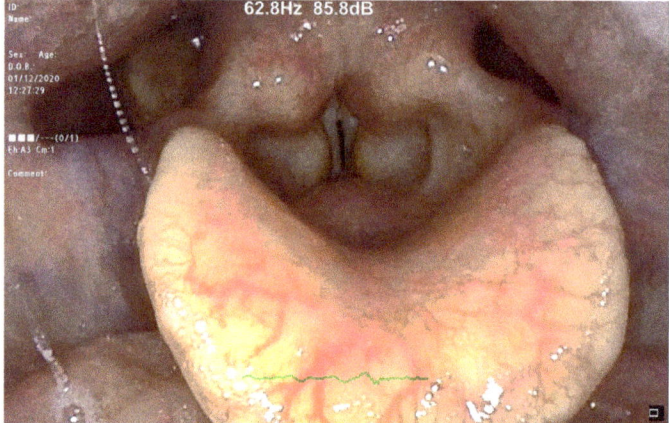

Figure CS.1. Muscle Tension Dysphonia image, displaying a distinct phonatory gap and compensatory compression of the false vocal folds. Image courtesy of Julian McGlashan, FRCS

Rehabilitation programme

Song Demonstrations

'Wanted Dead or Alive' (Bon Jovi); 'Like a Stone' and

'I'm the Highway' (Audioslave); 'Cascades of Gold' (Tide);

'Billie Jean' (Michael Jackson).

Session One

Song demonstration and plan of action
Overview of the laryngeal set up
Vocal hygiene
Establishing correct position and release of the jaw for open vowels
Siren to 'OO'
Singing section of a song to 'OO'

Session Two

Establishing jaw and mouth position for closed vowels
Optimising the siren 'OO'/'NG', incorporating vocal deconstriction
Introduction to breathing:
Low impact resistance to airflow (throat valve exercise)
Moderate impact resistance to airflow (finger valve exercise)

Session Three
- Revised breathing exercises from previous session
- Diaphragmatic function
- Pitched resistance to airflow - 'ZZ'

Session Four
- Pitched resistance to higher impact airflow - puffed cheeks
- Extension of finger valve exercise, working with the numerical table

Follow up sessions
- Revision of lip trill and 'OO' sirens
- Belting: Onsets
- Vocal Fry
- Promoting vocal economy and efficiency
- Maintaining vitality on inhale

Session One

Following an introductory chat, Ethan demonstrated his symptoms by singing a section of Bon Jovi's 'Wanted Dead or Alive'. His voice was cracking badly, particularly in the upper register, and the tone was very tight and strained. It was clear that he was driving the voice very hard and overblowing the sound, with high subglottic pressure. *"There are sensitive receptors to subglottic pressure levels below the vocal folds, and constant high pressure can cause dysphonia"* (Blake, Pers. Comm., 2020). Ethan's upper notes were inaccessible, and the constricted tone reflected his diagnosis. He admitted to being very uncomfortable, saying that he was experiencing a loss of confidence in his singing. I asked him to rate his demonstration, with 100% being the most comfortable, to which his response was 40%. In order to regain optimal voicing, I explained that we needed to explore the missing 60% and proposed a plan of action. This began with the importance of vocal hygiene, including hydration. Water is preferable for a singer to drink, as it helps lubrication of the vocal folds (especially the protective mucosal cover), allowing them to vibrate fully. It also provides moisture to the mouth and throat. Regular steam inhalation also improves hydration, but isn't recommended immediately before a gig, as the blood vessels dilate and come close to the surface of the vocal folds, potentially increasing the risk of haemorrhage.

I gave Ethan an overview of how the vocal mechanism works. Essentially, much like an inverted wind instrument (see Figure CS.2), vocal health is promoted when the various component parts and complex surrounding musculature are working in complete balance. He was also interested to see an image of healthy vocal folds (see Figure CS.3), enabling him to appreciate how this differed from a diagnosed MTD image. As with all clients, he was relieved to understand the physiological nature of his vocal pathology.

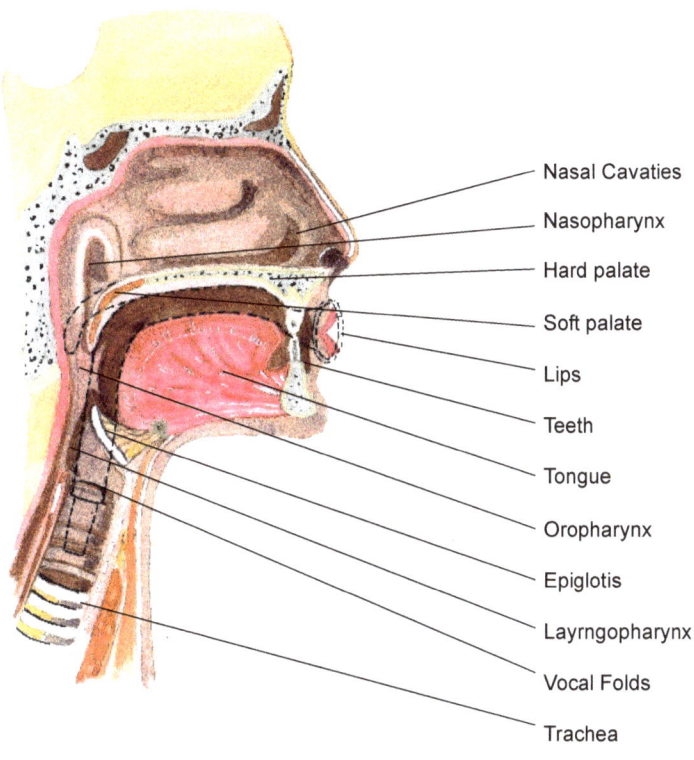

Figure CS.2. Cutaway of the vocal tract, with superimposed inverted wind instrument

Healthy Vocal Folds

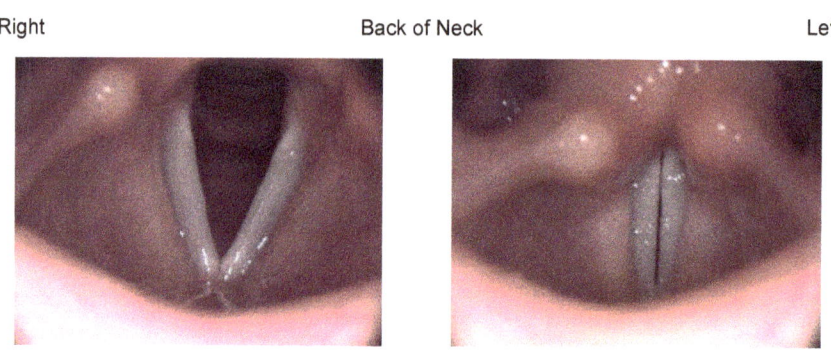

Figure CS.3. Stroboscopic images of healthy vocal folds.
Left image shows the folds ABducted, or apart.
Right image shows the folds ADducted, or together.

Jaw and mouth position for open vowels

Ethan had already mentioned that his breathing needed to be addressed, with which I readily agreed, but I decided to wait until the next session to tackle it. By now we were some way into the first session, and breathing requires more time in order to introduce it in the necessary detail. I had noticed some tension in his jaw when he was singing, which is normal where vocal constraint is present. By starting work on this aspect, I hoped that Ethan might experience an immediate sense of improved vocal wellbeing, even if only in a small way. Seeing a possible way forward in the initial stage of rehabilitation is crucial to regaining self-confidence.

Timeout: In touch with the TMJ

The temporomandibular joint (TMJ) is unique in that it is a bilateral joint that functions as one unit. Since it is connected to the mandible, the right and left joints on either side of the jaw must be mobilised together. '*By placing the fingers just in front of the small flap of skin in front of the ears and opening your mouth, you feel the head of the mandible (condoyle) moving forward and downwards to open up the mouth*' (Bunch Dayme 1995, pp.114–15). I encourage clients to recognise the feeling of this movement under their fingers like a 'bulge' when the mouth falls naturally into an oval shape and the chin is relaxed. Facial shape resembles an inverted triangle, with the base width being in line with the bulging jaw joints, and the raised cheekbones enhancing the angular lines leading down to the point of the chin. The muscles on either side of the mouth should be soft and disengaged. Forming the open vowels in this position can ease potential laryngeal tension and help to facilitate the appropriate tongue/palate relationship for accessing the full vocal harmonic spectrum.

If the jaw is pulled downwards only, without the forward movement of the mandible, it can put strain on the joint and interfere with the production of good vocal sound.

There can sometimes be psychological aspects that hinder the free and comfortable movement of the TMJ as, for example, a client who feels vulnerable with a more open mouth or thinks that it makes them look silly. However, they are generally convinced after I have demonstrated the position to them. I am always keen to point out that bone structure varies hugely from person to person, and that using the 'bulge' as a guideline can help to achieve appropriate release of the jaw and a mouth shape that is unique to each individual client. Once the 'bulge' is in place, it is important not to open the mouth any wider, as this can create tension in other parts of the vocal mechanism.

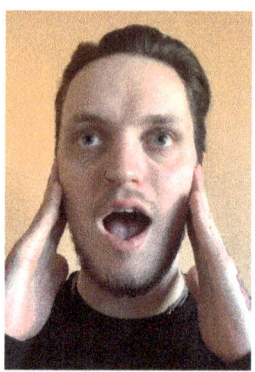

Figure CS.4. Jaw and mouth position for open vowels

Ethan was comfortable using a mirror to see, as well as feel, the bulging jaw joints rising beneath his fingers (Figure CS.4) - it is important for clients to become accustomed to using a mirror, as it acts as an extra sensory mechanism for helping to establish muscle memory. Still using the mirror for guidance, Ethan tried singing a lower section of the Bon Jovi song, keeping his fingers in place on the TMJ to maintain consistency of the jaw action on the open vowels, for example: 'bed' 'bad' 'bod' 'bored'. He was comfortable with his mouth being more open and rounded. Repeating the same passage away from the mirror, he began to experience a greater sense of vocal ease and flow that didn't compromise his integrity to the style of the song. To help consolidate consistency of movement and muscular flexibility, I asked him to sing the passage twice more.

Sirening (Pitch gliding) – 'OO'

In the second part of the session, I introduced Ethan to sirening (pitch gliding). This widely used technique acts as a barometer of vocal wellbeing and is a safe way to both warm up and warm down the voice, helping the larynx to return to its natural resting position after singing. It is a low impact exercise that can define vocal range and provide an easing effect on a voice that has been overused, especially over a substantial period of time. It enables gentle stretching and releasing of the vocal folds, revealing whether the crucial laryngeal action that controls this movement is functioning correctly. This action involves the paired crycothyroid muscles, which facilitate the tilting forward of the thyroid cartilage to allow lengthening and thinning of the vocal folds to access higher pitches. As a rehabilitator, my role is to discern whether long-standing tension has impacted adversely on the crycothyroid muscles, possibly causing the laryngeal tilt mechanism to malfunction. When I sense that could be the case, I will recommend some laryngeal physiotherapy before continuing rehabilitation (See footnote 1, p.16).

With its naturally rounded lip shape and high tongue position, I initially use an 'OO' vowel for sirening, as it is ideal for accessing acoustic resonance and upper harmonics. After demonstrating an 'OO' siren for him, Ethan made his first attempt. I encouraged him to envisage a rainbow along which he could direct the siren, not only to help it take wing and travel, but to emphasise forward momentum of the sound rather than a steep change of pitch. To underpin these factors and add vitality, I also asked him to imagine something joyful. Initially, his siren was rather bumpy and uneven, with some cracking as he went through the transition from the middle to high register on ascent and the middle to low register on descent. This is normal for a singer with MTD, as the mechanism is inevitably tight, and the high register of Ethan's voice had been inaccessible for some time. After repeating the siren twice more, he was experiencing a smoother transition through the vocal registers, and I was satisfied that I could continue without the need for laryngeal physiotherapy intervention.

The session ended with Ethan singing a complete song to 'OO'. To help facilitate vocal flow, he continued to maintain awareness of the 'OO' siren sensation and the idea of directing the notes of each phrase along an imaginary rainbow. As this vowel allows easier access to the head register, applying it to an entire song can help to ease muscular tension throughout its range and to gradually even out the register changes. Vocal registers, or register mechanisms, are differing patterns of vocal fold vibration. In order to strengthen the muscular 'set up' necessary for regaining high impact singing, vocal loading needs to be reduced throughout the vocal range. Hopefully, the lower and higher register mechanisms can begin to support each other, resulting in the strengthening of the middle register, which is so often undermined and weakened by the imbalance of the other two. The middle register can then gradually regain its role of acting as a bridge between the upper and lower registers. At this point, improved vocal wellbeing can often be glimpsed.

Ethan's choice of Audioslave's 'Like a Stone' worked well to 'OO'. His response to both the elements introduced in this session was positive and he left with a clear idea of what he needed to do to implement the given instructions. At various points I had referred to the necessity of establishing a systematic practice routine, providing details on the recording he had taken of the session.

Practice routine

Steam inhalation - up to ten minutes, initially three times a week and after a gig.

Jaw and mouth position for open vowels - using a mirror, establish the look and feel of the open vowels mouth shape by doing several jaw movements daily. Sing sections of songs with the fingers in front of the small flap of skin in front of the ears, so as to feel the 'bulge' of the jaw joints on the open vowels. Allow the sound to glide forward of its own accord. Repeat away from the mirror.

Sirens - do three 'OO' sirens twice daily, maintaining joy in the imagination. Incorporate two or three as a warm down after a gig.

Sing an entire song to 'OO' – envisaging each phrase being directed along a rainbow. Break the song into short sections, repeating each one several times until the voice is flowing smoothly and feeling comfortable.

Session Two

Ethan came for a second session a month later. Feedback and demonstration of all the previous session elements revealed that they had been successfully absorbed, as he could now replicate them optimally.

Jaw and mouth position for closed vowels

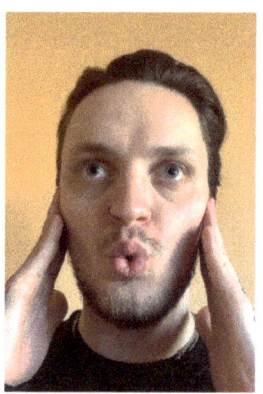

Figure CS.5. Jaw and mouth position for closed vowels

Having previously established the jaw and mouth position for open vowels, Ethan wanted to know how this differed from closed vowels, for example: 'boo' 'bid' 'bead'. I explained that the vowels in 'bid' and 'bead' should ideally be produced in the same shape as 'boo', with rounded rather than wide lips (Figure CS.5). This encourages a higher position of the tongue and soft palate, enabling easier access to a wider spectrum of acoustic energy. Using the mirror, he first pronounced a clear 'OO', and then slowly enunciated [i] (bid) and [ea] (bead) in as near the same mouth position as possible. Although noting that it felt rather unusual, he quickly perceived a greater sense of brightness in the tone of his voice. This perception remained as he added pitch, gently singing each of the words on a single note whilst maintaining the rounded mouth shape. He observed that the inverted triangular facial shape of the open vowels position remained, despite less prominence of the TMJ joints beneath his fingers. Further definition of the cheekbones was also noted, along with the crucial muscular stretch from each cheekbone down to the corners of the mouth (zygomatic muscles). Ethan noticed that both open and closed vowel positions maintained a rounded shape, pointing out that this concurred with the rounded bell of a wind instrument. Knowing that there are fundamentally only two choices of vowel shape for every sung syllable simplified the technical process for him, and he understood that these shapes need to be precisely actioned at the start of each beat in the music, unless there is a stylistic reason for not doing so.

Sirening (Pitch gliding) – 'NG', 'RR', 'ZZ', Lip trill

In the second part of this session, I continued to work with Ethan on his siren. I suggested that he try sirening to different sounds, starting with an 'NG'. Pronounced as in the word 'sing', this sound goes hand in hand with a sensation of the tongue rising upwards at the back of the mouth.

Using the mirror, we spent a few minutes setting up the position for an 'NG' siren. In order to recognise the contact between tongue and soft palate, it is best attempted in the open vowels jaw and mouth position. Being careful not to open his mouth any wider, which could compromise the necessary high tongue element, I asked Ethan to action the beginning of a yawn. He observed a lifting sensation at the back of the mouth, which I likened to creating an arch. After repeating this twice more, holding the muscular stretch for a few seconds each time, I asked him to repeat it again and try to locate the highest part of the arch, which I referred to as the 'keystone'. As he found this quite straightforward, I asked him to reset the position and try to stroke several 'NG' sounds across the 'keystone'. This produced a clear sensation of the tongue rising in the back of his mouth, and he was able to continue producing gently whining 'NG' sounds with increasingly clean onsets. He also began to recognise a sensation of nasal resonance. Ethan then tried a full 'NG' siren, maintaining the pitch as a continuous sensation of felt vibrations on the keystone. After a few attempts, his siren began to run smoothly across a wider vocal range, with the sound becoming increasingly more flowing and relaxed.

Timeout: The importance of 'NG'

'NG' is a velar consonant, in that it is articulated with the back (dorsum) of the tongue against the soft palate. Working with this sound begins the process of isolating and strengthening the different muscular actions of the tongue and soft palate, as it is vital that they can ultimately work together to maximise resonance and acoustic energy. Depending on the vocal genre, there will be occasions when a particular sound doesn't require such muscular precision. However, once acquired, a singer is in a position to exert personal choice, both to enhance versatility and to avoid limitation of a key aspect of vocal technique that may be required elsewhere. Mastering the tongue/soft palate relationship is also crucial to long term vocal health. With its high tongue position, the 'NG' sound blocks the air from the mouth cavity, excluding it as a resonator. This provides an opportunity for a higher head register to be experienced, often accompanied by a sensation of resonance behind the nose (by holding the nose in the middle of an 'NG' siren, it is possible to check that it is working properly as the sound should cut out). Nasal resonance is a very important aspect of singing, being associated with the 'ring' in the voice that invokes excitement in the listener due to its wide spectrum of acoustic energy. Working with an 'NG' siren helps to establish familiarity with nasal resonance, and also paves the way for the actioning of the soft palate that produces vowel sounds and clarity of vocal tone. The soft palate consists of an arched shape at the back of the mouth. Its elevation is most important in singing, as it creates more resonating space in the oropharynx and blocks off the nasopharynx (see Figure CS.2). The latter is crucial for the production of clear vowel sounds, and also prevents undesirable nasal tone. When working with 'NG', the soft palate is relaxed, with the uvula hanging down, referred to as an open nasal port. When it is elevated and blocking off the nasopharynx, it is referred to as a closed nasal port. The 'NG' high tongue position helps the soft palate to action nasal port closure, as this can only be optimally achieved if the tongue remains relatively high. Singers with significant tongue root tension (TRT) often have difficulty producing an 'NG', as they are unable to access the necessary high tongue position.

Ethan also enjoyed the increased sense of vitality that the 'RR', 'ZZ' and lip trill gave to his sirens. As he went from one to another, he experienced different core sensory perceptions, due to the subtle changes in breath pressure below the vocal folds that each sound promotes (see p.16). Able to roll an 'RR', he managed to maintain its rounded mouth shape throughout a siren, enabling maximum vocal economy and appropriate resistance to the air flow. After this, it was straightforward for him to apply the same rounded shape to the 'ZZ' siren, resulting in the same outcome. The 'ZZ' siren is a fricative consonant, being a voiced sound made by directing air through a small gap, that is, a semi-occluded vocal tract (see SOVT/Inertance p.36–37).

Because the mouth is partially closed, the increased variations of pressure are reflected back to the vocal folds, helping to balance the pressure from below (subglottic pressure) and allowing them to vibrate with greater ease and efficiency. Similarly, back pressure is returned to the vocal folds with lip trills, where the vibration of air is between the teeth and upper lip. There is a knack to achieving it, but he became more adept after a few attempts. To produce a successful lip trill, it is sometimes necessary to increase the tension of the upper lip by applying a gentle upward lift of the corners of the mouth with the forefingers. These four sirens enabled Ethan to focus on the sensation of creating sound vibration rather than on volume. *'It is thought that the primary benefit of SOVT exercises is to get the 'feel' of resonant voice, i.e., to get maximum sensory information about what is happening in the laryngeal vestibule in terms of energy conversion. Because acoustic pressures are maximum near occlusions, sensations should be felt in regions where the vocal tract area is small. Thus, for the bilabial fricative, one would expect strong vibrations to be sensed near the lips, teeth and the frontal part of the hard palate'* (Titze, 2001, p.525).

Optimising the siren - Laryngeal/vocal deconstriction

In order to fully optimise Ethan's siren, I wanted to eliminate potential laryngeal constriction in the higher range by introducing him to deconstriction. This would help to underpin the smooth transition through the registers on ascent and descent.

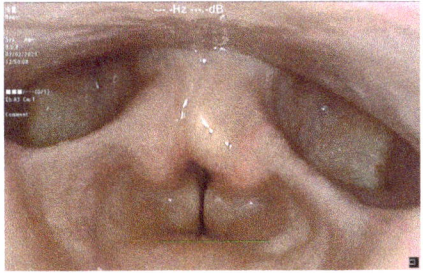

Figure CS.6. Laryngeal constriction. Image courtesy Julian McGlashan, FRCS

Timeout: Laryngeal constriction

Laryngeal constriction occurs when there is impingement of the false vocal folds (FVF) on the free movement of the true vocal folds (TVF), resulting in a tight and effortful sound. It is very common when there has been prolonged straining to reach high notes, particularly at a louder dynamic. This can cause excessive adduction (closure) of the TVF, much like a wind player overblowing the reed, producing typical symptoms of voice strain and potential muscle tension dysphonia (MTD). If left unaddressed, it can lead to vocal nodules. Deconstriction exercises help to address FVF tension, allowing the true vocal folds to access freedom of movement throughout the vocal range without being compromised. The FVF lie slightly above and to the sides of the TVF (see Figure CS.3). Between them is a small space called the laryngeal ventricle. Both sets of vocal folds act as valves to protect the airway and come together tightly when making forcing actions such as lifting, coughing and defecation. When voicing, however, the distance between the true and false vocal folds needs to be maintained. Laryngeal constriction can occur when the FVF begin to move across the TVF to the midline, compromising their freedom of movement (see Figure CS.6). There are two parts to vocal deconstriction exercises, both of which help to prevent FVF tension:

1) The FVF can be encouraged to retract by laughing silently, as inspired by Jo Estill's 'giggle' exercise (Estill, 1997). This helps to overcome untoward FVF constrictive and inward movement. The same effect can be achieved by whispering tenderly or making a very quiet laugh on *'ha ha'* from medium high to medium low in the pitch range (Shewell, 2009).

2) The second part uses the imagination to visualise an action that promotes a sense of width in the throat, for example: opening curtains/the expanding throat of a bullfrog/the widening neck of a cobra about to strike, helping to prevent FVF impingement on the true vocal folds.

Although deliberate constriction is used as an effect in some vocal styles, it is an advanced technique which needs to be used with full awareness of the potential risk to the vocal folds. In general, it is unlikely that singers can maintain full vocal health and longevity without the understanding and practical application of vocal deconstriction.

The following text is the conversation I (AMS) had with Ethan (E) about laryngeal deconstriction:

AMS: *"As you go higher, over the brow of the siren, would you agree that there is a perception that the vocal folds need something else to facilitate the flow of the siren at this point?"*

E: *"I get a sense of more pressure. It's not painful."*

AMS: *"That sense is the recognition of the increase of breath pressure, as these sounds provide an automatic resistance 'crutch' to the airflow. However, if you were singing normally and getting higher and louder, the voice could go one of two ways. It could either start to become strangulated with a feeling of constriction in the throat, as you have been experiencing, or you could do something to allow the vocal folds to accommodate the rising pitch and volume. This is the application of deconstriction, which ultimately enables the voice to find its own way to freedom. It is best introduced through the siren."*

E: *"That's good, because if I sing a phrase at the moment and I know there's a high note coming at the end, I find my body tensing up and I tend to throw my head back."*

AMS: *"Although tilting the head back is generally discouraged, there are times when it is thought to be appropriate, such as when belting. In this instance, it can help to accommodate the forward movement of the cricoid cartilage, allowing the vocal folds to remain shorter and thicker for higher notes. It is disputed as to whether this movement does takes place, but what is not in doubt is that the resulting sound is very loud and exciting when skilfully accomplished. It is thought that the unique belting volume level could come from the vocal folds adducting faster and for longer than in other singing styles."*

Ethan managed the deconstruction exercises well, relating to the idea of creating increased width at larynx level by visualising the action of curtains opening. After a couple of repetitions, he was rising to the challenge of maintaining width at larynx level without allowing the lips and mouth to widen as well. Being accustomed to using the effect of vocal distortion, which requires deliberate tonal constriction, Ethan understood the importance of mastering deconstruction in order to be able to distort his voice safely.

Siren setup

1. Direct the siren down an imaginary rainbow to encourage ease of vocal flow and colour. It translates readily into legato phrase shaping at a later stage.

2. Imagine a sense of joy and laughter to help vocal freedom and give intention to the sound.

3. Establish a rounded mouth shape for 'OO' and 'NG' sirens. Try to maintain this shape throughout the siren, and to avoid it from disintegrating.

4. Siren to lip trills, 'RR' (if accessible) and 'ZZ', to encourage higher breath pressure, engagement of the core and appropriate resistance to the airflow through the vocal folds.

5. Use an appropriate image to create width at larynx level on ascent, not only to prevent false vocal fold encroachment on the true vocal folds (laryngeal constriction), but also to allow the vocal tract to make subtle dimensional adjustments for accessing upper harmonics.

 Audio clip 4 – lip trill siren with deconstriction

Introduction to breathing

The remainder of the time was spent doing breath work, which is discussed fully in the preceding chapter. Referring to the inverted wind instrument analogy mentioned in the first session, I reiterated the principle that the vocal folds act as a valve and function as a double reed. In order to prevent further vocal strain, I explained that there needs to be a clear distinction between overblowing the reed and achieving appropriate airflow through it. Although Ethan's vocal style of high impact belting required the equivalent of a large diesel engine, it relied on fine muscular tuning as well as strength. The first step to achieving this was to encourage a more gentle muscular engagement.

Before starting with the throat valve breathing exercise (see p.31–34), I referred to the analogy of two balloons to describe differing lung function (see Balloon A and Balloon B, p.28-29). Having explained the benefit of doing this exercise in a prone position, Ethan was happy to try it lying on his back. I outlined the idea of creating low airflow resistance through the vocal folds on both exhalation and inhalation, stressing the importance of equalising the length of both whilst maintaining a consistent level of pressure. After some initial qualms about not being able to access enough air, he found it relaxing and accessible, with the perception of the abdominal rise and fall being primarily in the navel area. As this movement gradually became more even and rhythmic, I began counting to help him establish an equal exhale/inhale ratio of approximately 4:4 seconds. In order to achieve maximum benefit, it is necessary to follow this up in practice with 6–12 perfectly balanced breaths.

Before coming back to standing, I asked Ethan to do a few more breaths. This time I asked him to maintain the throat breathing 'HAH' sound on the exhale, but relinquish it on the inhale, opening his mouth instead and waiting to see what happened:

E: *"I can feel the navel rising in the same way."*

Letting go of the instinctive impulse to actively engage with the inhalation had allowed his respiratory system to assimilate a deeper breathing pattern.

Being physically fit and having responded well to the first breathing exercise, I decided to introduce Ethan to the second one straightaway. Based on the same principle, it involves greater resistance to the airflow and uses the forefingers to emulate the vocal folds (see Finger Valve

Breathing Exercise on p.35–40). In his high impact CCM singing, Ethan had got into a habitual pattern of excessive core engagement. Having now experienced low level engagement in the throat breathing exercise, I wanted him to experience it at a moderate level. Over time, this would enable gradual development of deeper core strength, allowing recognition of the appropriate muscular engagement required to achieve his vocal goals in a safe and long-lasting way.

Ethan quickly mastered the finger valve breathing, immediately recognising deeper abdominal engagement on exhalation. Due to the presence of airflow resistance at a higher level, inhalation in this exercise is more challenging. Instruction has to be given with caution, as it can lead to tension in the abdomen if the muscles are not sufficiently developed. Because of his fitness level, I decided to let him try it. On exhalation, he could sense a more sequential muscular engagement, feeling the deeper internal obliques (IO) coming into play towards the end of the breath. On inhalation, he was able to feel the crucial disengagement of these muscles, along with the observation that there was no upward lift of his shoulders (see Blake, Pers. Comm., 2020 on p.25, *"If the obliques remain constantly engaged..."*). As with the first exercise, I advised an equal exhale/inhale ratio of approximately 4:4 seconds, stressing the importance of limiting this more strenuous exercise to four breaths in total. I also pointed out the importance of being aware that these two breathing exercises were intended purely to build muscular stamina and once achieved, would be applied to singing in a later session.

Practice routine

Closed vowels - using the mirror, speak the closed vowels 'boo' 'bid' 'bead', maintaining a rounded 'OO' mouth shape. When this feels comfortable, add pitch by gently singing each one on a single note. Repeat several times a week.

Siren – continue using the different sounds on a regular basis for ongoing vocal health, and as part of both vocal warm up and warm down.

Throat valve breathing exercise – gradually establish an equal exhale/inhale ratio of approximately 4:4 seconds. In order to achieve maximum benefit, try to follow this up with 6-12 perfectly balanced breaths. Practise daily to begin with, and then as feels comfortable on an ongoing basis. It is effective after strenuous vocal activity and when experiencing stress, as it has a calming effect on the nervous system.

Finger valve breathing exercise – introduce daily, when the above breathing exercise has been comfortably assimilated. Proceed with caution, maintaining an exhale/inhale 4:4 seconds ratio at a moderate and consistent pressure. Limit to four breaths only. It is best not to be attempted when feeling tired or physically debilitated.

Session Three

When Ethan returned for a third session six weeks later, it was apparent that he had made significant progress, having put a lot of dedicated time into his practice. He accurately demonstrated both the breathing exercises, with evidence of a more subtle muscular response. His systematic approach was clearly beginning to bear fruit. I felt it appropriate at this point to reinforce the exercises by explaining diaphragmatic function, explaining its relevance and importance in singing (see Regulating diaphragmatic action in singing, p.48). Ethan was happy to take more time to fully understand the mechanics of breathing.

Having shown him illustrations of the diaphragm (see Figures 1, 2 and 5) I guided him through a practical demonstration.

AMS: *"We start by interlocking the fingers and creating a dome shape with the hands, which represents the diaphragm. As we breathe in, the hands lower into a flat position as the ribs expand. As we breathe out, the hands return to the dome shape as the lungs deflate. This replicates the action of the diaphragm in everyday breathing, as in the Balloon A analogy I gave you in the last session. The diaphragm plays a vital part in achieving optimal vocal function but, being a muscle that is not completely under our conscious control, I refer to it as the 'puppet' muscle. You have experienced abdominal movement in the breathing exercises, and it is this muscular area that I refer to as the 'puppeteer', having vital attachments to the diaphragm which influence its rise and fall. In order to lengthen the breath and be able to sustain the voice safely and consistently, this action has to be modified for singing. The abdominal muscles are key to this modification and mastering the breathing exercises will enable you to achieve it."*

E: *"Ok".*

AMS: *"When you started the throat valve breathing exercise, you were a little panicky at first, due to feeling short of breath and wanting to gasp in the air. This is a normal reaction, which will become clear as we now use the hands in a different way to demonstrate the action of the diaphragm when singing. This corresponds to last session's Balloon B analogy. Starting again with the hands in a dome shape, we breathe in as before, lowering them into a flattened position as the ribs expand. This time we breathe out through pursed lips, introducing resistance to the airflow and activating a different diaphragmatic response, with the hands now rising much slower. The increase in breath pressure exerts a brake effect on the ascent of the diaphragm, preventing it from collapsing upwards so quickly. However, with the 'fight and flight' survival mechanism being so deeply ingrained, taking an in breath when the diaphragm has only partially ascended can give rise to a feeling of panic. Singers have to learn how to override this sensation and become accustomed to the breath being topped up whilst the lungs still contain air. By maintaining the valve on inhale in the breathing exercises, the diaphragm is encouraged to lower whilst in its upward ascent, allowing the air that has been expelled on the preceding exhale to top up automatically."*

E: *"So it's fine to breathe like that when singing?"*

AMS: *"Yes – it's essential."*

E: *"Weird!"*

AMS: *"If you breathe in by gasping the air and raising the shoulders, the subsequent exhale is going to be quite short and quick, as there is no valve in place to regulate the breath pressure. Rapid collapse of the ribs and lungs on exhale is inevitably followed by another gasping inhale. It is vocally dangerous to belt when breathing in this way, as the vocal folds rely on a higher breath pressure beneath them to support that amount of vocal load. Without the appropriate subglottic pressure in place when singing high and loud, there will inevitably be compensatory muscle movement of the surrounding musculature which is what leads to MTD and the symptoms you have experienced. Singers and wind players have to establish an alternative way to harness the breath, in order to activate the vocal folds/reed efficiently. Once the 'fight and flight' response has been overridden, the diaphragm can more readily engage with the automatic topping up of air on inhalation."*

E: *"And that's how we fit it into phrases when we're singing."*

AMS: *"Yes. Through the exercises, I'm teaching you how to breathe in before you've finished breathing out. It is important to first master the exhale/inhale 4:4 ratio, because slowing the inhale helps to train the diaphragm to respond more readily to descend whilst in the process of ascent. As this response strengthens, the ratio can be modified, allowing you to take quicker breaths without unbalancing the vocal mechanism. I will introduce you to this in the next session, by using a numerical modification table."*

E: *"OK. For now, I've got to reinforce the equal ratio in the muscle memory."*

AMS: *"Yes. This is how I've worked with clients on breathing issues over a long period, gradually honing and refining the technique to make it completely suitable for purpose."*

E: *"Brilliant."*

AMS: *"You'll do this, and once you've got there, you'll stay there. You will achieve the vocal health and longevity that you need, despite the vocal challenges that your high impact singing style demands. It's like doing a sprint all the time. Although asking a lot, once you have complete balance of the whole mechanism, the voice will and can do it! Do you have any questions?"*

E: *"No. I just need to go through the recording a few times for it to sink in."*

Now that the preparation was complete regarding breath work, I wanted to apply it to singing as soon as possible.

Much like the breathing exercises, this had to be done in stages, gradually leading Ethan back to high impact singing by starting with a more gentle approach. In my own singing studies, I learnt a technique that suited this purpose ideally, which I continue to use for maintaining my own voice and vocal wellbeing.

AMS: *"Let's leave the big singing for the moment. I'm going to teach you now how to apply the valve principle to pitched sound, having successfully mastered it in the breathing exercises. For this we use 'ZZ', as in the siren from last session. It is a fricative consonant, which is a voiced sound made by directing air through a small gap, and its pronunciation involves the vibration of the vocal folds. Applying it to a melody is a unique way of achieving the precise abdominal engagement for any pitch in any song. As with the siren, the lips need to be rounded to maximise full vocal economy. Before trying it to a melody, it's best to start by pursing the lips and breathing out for about four seconds. This should create a hissing sound as the air is released through the small aperture. It is a knack, requiring about 50% effort and moderate pressure, resulting in automatic core engagement as the appropriate level of resistance to the* airflow through the vocal folds is established.... That's it! Now, keeping the same rounded mouth position, breathe out to a spoken 'ZZ'. It's like the buzzing sound of an electric shaver, and you can sense the teeth playing a part in resisting the airflow."

E: "Ok".

AMS: "That's it. You feel just fractional abdominal engagement?"

E "Yes. Not as much as in the breathing exercises."

AMS: "No, but you can sense it. If you repeat the 'ZZ', you will hear that it actually creates a low-pitched note.... Good! Now I'm going to demonstrate a few notes to the 'ZZ' sound.... It's like becoming a wind player, with the buzzing 'ZZ' being equivalent to the mouthpiece. This activates the reed which, in a singer's case, is in the throat and not attached to the mouthpiece. Using the 'ZZ', see if you can sound those notes as I did, as if you're blowing them through the vocal reed.... Excellent! Because of the changing pitch, there is a corresponding change in breath pressure and airflow, causing the degree of abdominal engagement to adjust accordingly. As long as the 'ZZ' is maintained optimally, with a clearly audible buzzing *sound and no collapse of the mouth position, you will feel a deeper engagement on the higher notes which, crucially, happens automatically. There should be a corresponding sensation of energy and vitality being harnessed within the core."*

E: *"Yes. It's good that the engagement adjusts for higher notes. Maybe it's because of the change in vocal fold vibration?"*

AMS: *"Yes. Which is why the appropriate diaphragmatic action is vital, as it plays a key role in regulating that vibration."*

The session continued with Ethan singing a section of 'I'm the Highway' (Audioslave) to 'ZZ'. He was able to recognise the abdominal release synchronising with his inhale, which he noticed was becoming increasingly automatic. However, he needed to take longer between phrases in order for this to happen, at the same time becoming accustomed to the inhale being topped up by mouth. Gradually, he overcame the instinct to consciously pull the air in!

E: *"Sometimes I want to snap a bit of air in first."*

AMS: *"Yes, but try not to give in to that response. Wanting to gasp in the air is an instinctive reaction when learning to allow the diaphragm to descend whilst in its upward ascent."*

E: *"Yes, that's how it feels, and when I just wait between phrases for the navel release to happen, it does do it!"*

AMS: *"Excellent."*

After repeating the song section to 'ZZ', Ethan found himself releasing a substantial amount of residual air. I pointed out that this happens because the lungs retain some air when using the breath in this way.

Continuing with the 'ZZ', I suggested repeating the same section up to three times when practising. Starting with a small number of phrases would enable the new breathing pattern to be assimilated, and at the same time encourage the muscles to start patterning themselves optimally to that sequence of notes. In order to underpin efficacy of the breath and vocal economy, I asked Ethan to try, where possible, to maintain a rounded mouth shape between phrases.

Finally, I asked him to sing the song section to the words, explaining that when the 'ZZ' is removed and the mouth opens for normal singing, the action of the abdomen should stay exactly the same. Being mindful of the inhale, Ethan's first attempt was very heartening:

Audio clip 5 – segment from 'I'm the Highway' after working it to 'ZZ'

I ended the session by thanking him for his ready response and willingness to learn, acknowledging that his patience and acceptance of instruction made it easier for me to help him. This is exemplified by the following clip, taken from Ethan's final session, when his work with 'ZZ' was fully optimised:

 Audio clip 6 – segment from 'Billie Jean' to 'ZZ'

Practice routine

Breathing – continue to maintain the Session 2 exercises.

Preparation for 'ZZ' exercise – make an 'OO' mouth shape and breathe out in this position to a 'ZZ' sound. This should produce a steady buzz as it triggers moderate resistance to the airflow, accompanied by a sensation of gentle abdominal engagement. Observe that the 'ZZ' creates a pitched note.

Pitched 'ZZ' – sustain a few single notes to 'ZZ', then experiment with short sequences of notes, gradually spreading out in both directions from a mid-range starting point. Aim to maintain a clearly audible buzzing sound, with no collapse of the mouth position as the pitch changes. Be sure not to trigger vocal discomfort or constraint by getting too close to vocal range extremities.

Song to 'ZZ' – sing a middle range song section to a smooth 'ZZ', allowing the contours of the phrases to be shaped by the buzzing sound. Try to observe how abdominal release begins to synchronise with the inhale. Repeat until comfortable, and then move on to the next section.

Song with lyrics – sing the song with the words, observing that abdominal engagement should remain the same as when using 'ZZ'.

Session Four

I was aware that much of Ethan's rehabilitation so far had focused on breath management. However, in order for him to gain full mastery over his high impact vocal style, there remained one essential aspect to cover. This was to apply the valve principle to a second pitched sound, with the aim of generating the necessary muscular effort needed for safe singing at this level. Made by directing air through a smaller aperture, this sound is also voiced, but unlike 'ZZ' it isn't a fricative consonant. It is referred to as 'puffed cheeks', where the cheeks are filled with air which is then directed through the small aperture made by the lips (see SOVT and Inertance p.36–37). Requiring more effort and higher breath pressure than 'ZZ', it remains similar in that there is automatic engagement of the core as the appropriate level of resistance to the airflow through the vocal folds comes into play. The difference when working with 'puffed cheeks' is that the air resistance level is significantly higher. As with 'ZZ', Ethan began by creating the shape and exhaling through it. He was quick to observe that abdominal engagement was stronger, as the air passing through the lips was under greater pressure and producing a high intensity hissing sound. Following the same procedure as 'ZZ', he used this technique to sing single notes followed by short melodic fragments. He described the sensation of pitching notes as slightly ethereal, saying that he was mainly aware of them as sound vibrations above the hissing sound of the breath. Another observation was of feeling a much stronger core engagement when pitching notes in this way. I was interested to see how his body would accommodate the stronger abdominal inhale when working with higher breath pressure sound.

AMS: *"The inhale here is more challenging, as it requires greater precision to achieve the necessary exhale/inhale balance when engaging and disengaging deeper muscular abdominal layers. You are now familiar with the inhale release, but with this higher impact work you can't as yet achieve a sufficiently deep release when taking quick breaths between phrases."*

E: *"Right. Yes."*

AMS: *"Even when using a microphone, singing at a higher pressure still requires a corresponding level of muscular activity on inhale. In other words, the higher pressure singing inevitably results in activation of the deeper abdominal muscular layers, which crucially have* to be switched off between phrases…. and you've got to be able do this quickly."

E: "Yes, definitely."

AMS: "In order to acquire the skill of balancing a long exhale with a quick, powerful inhale, you need to start by using the puffed cheeks like an airflow 'crutch' for the exhale."

E: "I can really feel engagement in the core with the puffed cheeks."

AMS: "Good. When you're blowing high and loud notes through tighter pursed lips, the body itself will work out the appropriate muscular engagement. If you work a song in this way, doing it to puffed cheeks two or three times, you are laying down the pattern of how much your abdominal 'throttle' has to engage. That's what rehabilitation is all about, in that you learn to avoid over or under muscular engagement. Essentially, you would use the puffed cheeks technique to prepare all your high impact songs. With lower impact ones, it's better to use a lower impact airflow 'crutch' such as 'ZZ'."

E: "Yes. That makes sense."

AMS: *"Let's try that section again with puffed cheeks. Would you do it twice, waiting in between phrases to fully allow and recognise the sensation of deeper core release."*

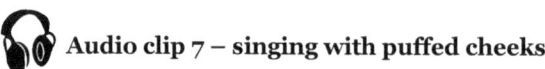 **Audio clip 7 – singing with puffed cheeks**

AMS: *"That's excellent. Now I have to give you the extension to the finger valve exercise that we started in Session 2. It should enable you to achieve the deeper core release more quickly, in order to shorten inhale time."*

E: *"Yes. That's a struggle for me. I have nearly passed out sometimes because of holding the core really tight and carrying on and on singing."*

AMS: *"That is the nub of all this work. Having lain down the muscular pattern of how much your abdominal 'throttle' has to engage when singing, you now have to pattern the muscles for it to disengage when not singing. If you can't achieve full abdominal release between phrases in the appropriate amount of time before starting to sing again, you will inevitably default to 'fight and flight' breathing and a gasping inhale."*

I took Ethan through the extension of the finger valve exercise, for which I use a numerical table as a guide to progressive inhale shortening (see Figure 4 and audio clip 'Working with the numerical table', p.40–41. He responded well, understanding that it is a standalone exercise which should automatically have a knock-on effect to singing as the muscles begin to release quicker on the back of it. I demonstrated the 4:1 ratio final section of the table, explaining that the sensation by that time is of a powerful, muscular swingback action when inhaling quickly.

AMS: *"Try working with puffed cheeks for your higher impact singing, initially taking time over the inhale to effect a deep release. Once you've worked through the numerical table, you will find that the inhale automatically starts to quicken when singing, giving an accompanying sensation of muscular vigour. You then remove the puffed cheeks airflow 'crutch' and sing the song normally, when the muscular patterning of both exhale and inhale should stay in place. That brings us full circle from when you said in our first session that you knew you were overbreathing."*

E: *"Yes. Spot on. Fantastic."*

Practice routine

Preparation for 'puffed cheeks' exercise – puff out the cheeks and blow a steady stream of air through the small aperture made by the lips. Abdominal engagement should feel significantly stronger than the 'ZZ' exhale, with the airstream producing a high intensity hissing sound.

Using 'puffed cheeks' to produce pitch – begin by sustaining a few single notes, and then experiment with short melodic fragments. The sensation when pitching notes in this way is mainly an awareness of them vibrating above the hissing of the breath, which can be felt on the palm of the hand. Repeat note sequences several times in order to establish abdominal muscle memory patterning.

Finger valve exercise extension – work through the numerical table as a guide to progressive inhale shortening. This is a standalone exercise, which has a knock-on effect to singing, especially when taking quick breaths. Abdominal muscular sensation should gradually become that of a powerful, swing back action.

Although he had completed the four recommended sessions, it had been necessary to spend a lot of time regulating Ethan's breath function, and there were other rehabilitative techniques that I wanted to cover. I enquired about the possibility of seeing him again, to which he agreed, returning four more times over the next fourteen months. By this time, he had successfully assimilated the breath work and was able to re-access his upper range without discomfort. He could now comfortably sustain longer passages with more power and a greater feeling of confidence.

Follow up sessions

Revision of lip trill and 'OO' sirens

For ongoing flexibility and evenness across his full range, I stressed the importance of continuing to gauge vocal wellbeing by monitoring sirening function, adding that the siren can be used on all vowels. I also pointed out that it was essential to keep singing songs to 'OO' as well as to lyrics, being careful to maintain both its rounded shape and the muscular sensation of stretch from the TMJ to the corners of the mouth. Playing a vital role in addressing vocal loading issues, singing belting passages to 'OO' allows the different laryngeal movement for each sound to be actioned on the same melodic section. It is crucial to be able to accommodate the changes in vocal fold length and thickness that each movement provides, and to have equal access to both for ongoing vocal wellbeing. Ultimately, this leads to increased laryngeal muscular compatibility and stamina.

 Audio clip 8 – lip trill siren

 Audio clip 9 – 'OO' siren

 Audio clip 10 – revision of 'Like a Stone' to 'OO'

 Audio clip 11 – revision of 'Like a Stone' with lyrics

Belting

E: *"What I tend to do in preparation for the high impact singing is to lightly sing a song backstage and gently ease myself into it. I'll sing the higher passages an octave lower to begin with or sing a harmony around the melody until my voice begins to feel flexible and comfortable. I also sing sections of the songs I'm about to perform to 'OO' and 'ZZ' to make sure that I'm fully limbered up vocally. Regarding belting, I've realised now that what sounds good and feels comfortable when recording is very different to singing at a gig. There are three songs that I belt the whole way through in performance. It doesn't blow my voice, but it really tires me out."*

AMS: *"It's like a continuous vocal sprint."*

E: *"Yes, I know that now."*

The technique of belting is widely documented and can be read elsewhere. My focus with Ethan was to clarify the way in which the vocal folds are employed when belting, in that they remain shorter and thicker on higher notes as opposed to transitioning to lengthening and thinning at the point of handover to the upper register. Because the vocal folds adduct for longer on each vibratory cycle, the potential for overload and damage is high if a singer isn't sufficiently aware of these differences. It is easy to incur unwanted constriction, but this can be overridden by learning how to create the appropriate vocal loading for every note of a song. Ethan was now fully competent regarding airflow management, to which I added further anchoring techniques to accommodate the high levels of effort required in the head, neck and torso when belting.

Glottal onset

Although a natural belter, relying largely on instinct prior to his diagnosis, Ethan needed more information regarding the initiation of tone. Glottal onset is a recognised belting technique. It involves the build-up of moderate breath pressure beneath closed vocal folds prior to voicing, resulting in a clicking noise as they gently explode apart when the sound starts. Conversely, if the breath precedes the tone (aspirate onset), not only can it prevent the required closure of the vocal folds needed for safe belting, but it can also potentially cause trauma in this high impact vocal quality. Following on from the laryngeal deconstriction work in Session

2, I suggested that Ethan substitute the 'silent giggle' sensation with inwardly high crying, or 'silent screaming', in order to raise the breath pressure beneath the vocal folds and encourage sufficient retraction of the false vocal folds prior to attempting the onset. This would also help to maintain a high larynx, another component of belting physiology.

Having mastered the 'silent screaming' sensation, Ethan used the sound 'UH-OH' to create the glottal onset. I asked him to briefly hold the sensation of pressure beneath the larynx before voicing to ensure sufficient false vocal fold retraction. After a few attempts his onsets became cleaner with easier projection, and he could sense the gentle 'click' at the start of the sound. He was gradually able to match the dynamic level of the onset with that of the dynamic necessary for belting. He also tried 'EH-OH' and 'AA-OH' onsets, observing that *"The pressure has to be there beforehand, but not too much, as I sense it could lead to constriction."*

Onsetting lyrics in speech and singing

Using the lyrics 'Awakened, back to the beginning' (Cascade of Gold), Ethan practised the initial 'A' as a glottal onset. Then, using the same technique, he 'onsetted' each syllable separately, aiming at an imaginary target on the other side of the room. When comfortable with that, I asked him to think of placing the pitch of each note on the target, to which he could then throw the sung syllables, with the intent of both consonant and vowel being on the same pitch.

 Audio clip 12 – onsetting lyrics in speech and singing

The next step was to make the transition from onsets to straight singing. This incorporates the simultaneous onset (breath and tone at the same time), which is the main feature of classical singing. In belting, however, the first step is to achieve a good glottal onset, which leads on to safe simultaneous onsets, as the high degree of effort in pitch preparation can then be assured.

 Audio clip 13 – transitioning from onsets to straight singing

I also encouraged Ethan to practice onsets to 'Y' (yellow), which help to mobilise a high-sided tongue action. This creates the higher dorsum position necessary for belting.

There was a six-week gap between Sessions 5 and 6, during which Ethan became more confident with onsets:

 Audio clip 14 – sustained pitch onsets

 Audio clip 15 – onsetting pitched lyrics of complete phrase

Vocal fry

Ethan began to comment on how the different technical elements we had covered during his rehabilitation process were now beginning to weld together. On one occasion, when we were discussing the benefits of extending the siren to the bottom of the voice, especially when warming down after a gig, he mentioned vocal fry:

"I like the feeling of vocal fry. I do it quite a lot, including when I'm gigging."

The vocal fry register (also known as creak, croak, glottal fry, glottal scrape) is the lowest vocal register and is produced through a loose glottal closure that permits air to bubble through the vocal folds slowly with a popping or rattling sound of a very low frequency (Chapman, 2006, p.67). Like any other vocal register, the vocal fry register has a unique vibratory pattern of the vocal folds. In some cases, vocal pedagogues have found the use of vocal fry therapeutically helpful to students who have trouble producing lower notes. Singers often lose their low notes or never learn to produce them because of the excessive tension of the laryngeal muscles and of the support mechanism that leads to too much breath pressure (Greene and Mathieson, 2001).

Promoting vocal economy and efficiency

Rounding the 'EE' vowel - although not necessary to maintain a consistently rounded 'EE', it is helpful to be able to produce it in this shape (see Figure CS.5). As well as encouraging elevation of the back of the tongue to access upper harmonics, it also helps to prevent the sides of the mouth from pulling back, which can trigger tongue retraction.

Pitching consonants – in the rock/pop genre, there can be a conflict between remaining true to the style and achieving vitality in both tone and lyrics. Using a microphone can lull singers into weak articulation, especially in the low to middle range. However, it is particularly important to make the beginnings of words clear and vital in order to maintain vocal energy. Having touched on consonants when onsetting song lyrics, Ethan was receptive to doing more consonant specific work. This will be covered in greater detail in other client case studies in later volumes.

 Audio clip 16 – consonant work and rounding the 'EE' vowels

E: *"It definitely feels as if using consonants in this way to project my voice helps to detract from the emphasis on how my voice sounds."*

AMS: *"Cleanly projected consonants encourage the tongue to be more flexible, allowing it to make the minute adjustments between each vowel to access full vocal colour. It's a good exercise for maximising compatibility of the articulators (tongue, teeth and lips), as it helps to alleviate vocal tension by limiting vocal fold load."*

Tongue work – having a flexible tongue is essential in maximising vocal efficiency. Tongue root tension (TRT) is a common problem for singers, and often compromises freedom in other parts of the mechanism. Wanting to capitalise on the 'EE' vowel and consonant work, Ethan rose well to the challenges of specific tongue flexibility exercises. Working with TRT will be covered in greater detail in other client case studies in later volumes in this series.

Maintaining vitality on inhale

AMS: *"When you are accustomed to releasing the breath in the core, it harnesses a sensation of vitality in the navel area between phrases. This adds overall impact to the song, as it allows an audience to remain engaged in your performance. Whatever the mood of the lyrics, the silence between phrases needs to remain vital in order to transmit the thought from one phrase to the next."*

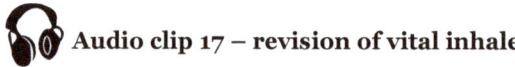

Audio clip 17 – revision of vital inhale

AMS: *"It's also essential to master a springback, rather than a passive muscular action, when inhaling quickly."*

Audio clip 18 – revision of springback inhale

Seven months passed between Ethan's penultimate and final session. This gave him the opportunity to become more vocally self-reliant. Before being discharged, it is necessary for clients to start to take responsibility for the management of their ongoing vocal health. Over the months, he had been accumulating and assimilating the techniques that allowed him to master this crucial part of the rehabilitation process. I asked him how he felt now about the efficacy of breathing and the need as a singer to be a vocal athlete:

 Audio clip 19 – benefits of breathing on vocal health

AMS: *"Before runners do a sprint, they spend a long time leading up to it by limbering and warming up. It's similar to yoga. Before doing the very demanding postures, it's necessary to prepare in a specific way. That's what you need to remember for your future vocal health!"*

E: *"Yes definitely"*.

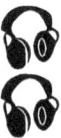 Audio clip 20 – maintenance of vocal longevity

Audio clip 21 – utilising the full potential of the vocal folds

Audio clip 22 – customised singing exercises

By the end of this session, all aspects of Ethan's rehabilitation process had been revised and clarified. He finished by singing 'Billie Jean', demonstrating both his return to vocal health and his ability to provide the full performance package:

 Audio clip 23 – extract from 'Billie Jean' marriage of music and lyrics

Outcome

Throughout his rehabilitation, it had been important to create a sense of teamwork with Ethan, as I needed to help him remedially whilst at the same time respecting his vocal genre. Although painstaking work, he had successfully learnt to take control of his voice and, also, how to deal with it on the inevitable vocal 'down days'. He was now singing comfortably throughout his range with a sound technique and could begin to enjoy performing again with new-found confidence. He understood that it was necessary to rotate all his exercises on an ongoing basis to effect vocal longevity, and to be the means by which he could fully trust his voice in performance.

Whilst Ethan's rehabilitation process may give hope to others with the same diagnosis, it is important to stress that each case is unique. It is by no means assured that the same course of action would necessarily result in the same outcome.

Youtube clips

The Cardigans – Favourite Game
(EC Acoustic Cover)

https://www.youtube.com/watch?v=q8NPV8DKKIE
(Accessed 27 May 2021)

Matt Corby – Brother
(EC Acoustic Cover)

https://www.youtube.com/watch?v=Y4MpziSKxv4
(Accessed 27 May 2021)

Ethan Cronin – Cascades of Gold.
Recorded a month after the last rehabilitation session.

https://www.youtube.com/watch?v=GmnB6nugFC0
(Accessed 27 May 2021)

"My sessions with Alison were essential to me, and really opened my eyes to the way the whole body works to create vocal sound. I was heading down a dark path, in which I could have completely blown my voice permanently and ruined my career. This was due to my lack of knowledge about how sound is actually produced. The rehabilitation sessions have really kicked off my career as a session vocalist and, with my new understanding of the voice, I haven't had a problem since. It's essential to know how I'm making the sound and how to use it correctly to get the best results, including how to practise. Alison was amazing, and I always recommend her to any vocalists who are having trouble or need to understand the science behind the voice." - Ethan

References

Brown, Oren L. (1996) *Discover Your Voice – How to Develop Healthy Voice Habits.* San Diego, CA: Singular Publishing Group, Inc.

Bunch Dayme, Meribeth (1995) *Dynamics of the Singing Voice* 3ed. Wien, New York, NY: Springer-Verlag.

Calais-Germain, Blandine and Germain, François (2016) *Anatomy of Voice.* Rochester, VT: Healing Arts Press.

Chapman, Janice L. (2006) *Singing and Teaching Singing, A Holistic Approach to Classical Voice.* San Diego, CA: Plural Publishing, Inc.

Estill, Jo (1997) *Estill Voice Training System Level One: Compulsory Figures for Voice Control.* Pittsburg, PA: Estill Voice Training Systems.

Goldsack, Christopher (2019) Physics of the Voice. Presentation at AOTOS Summer Conference, Woodland Grange, Leamington Spa, 19–21 July.

Greene and Mathieson (2001) *The Voice and Its Disorders* 6ed. London: Whurr.

Morris, Ron (2014) Breathing - Accent Method. Presentation at AOTOS South West Study Day, Tiverton, UK, March.

Hixon, Thomas J. (2006) *Respiratory Function in Singing.* Tucson, AZ: Redington Brown.

Hodges, P.W. and Gandevia, S.C. (2000) Changes in intra-abdominal pressure during postural and respiratory activitation of the human diaphragm. *Journal of Applied*

Physiology (1985) 89(3):967–76. https://journals.physiology.org/doi/full/10.1152/jappl.2000.89.3.967 (Accessed 27 May 2021)

Miller, Richard (1986) *The Structure of Singing*. New York, NY: Schirmer Books.

Myers, Thomas W. (2014) *Anatomy Trains: Myofascial Meridians for Manual and Movement Therapists* 3ed. Edinburgh: Churchill Livingstone.

Ramaswami, Srivatsa (2000) *Yoga for the Three Stages of Life: Developing your Practice as an Art Form, a Physical Therapy, and a Guiding Philosophy*. Rochester, VT: Inner Traditions International.

Shewell, Christina (2009) *Voice Work*. Oxford: Wiley-Blackwell.

Svec, Jan G., Schutte, Harm K., Chen, C. Julian, Titze, Ingo R. (2021) Integrative insights into the myoelastic-aerodynamic theory and acoustics of phonation. Scientific tribute to Donald G. Miller. *Journal of Voice*. https://doi.org/10.1016/j.jvoice.2021.01.023.

Titze, Ingo R. (2001) Acoustic interpretation of resonant voice. *Journal of Voice* 15(4):519–28.

Titze, Ingo R. (2011) The affect of epilarynx tube dimensions on glottal airflow. *The Journal of the Acoustical Society of America* 130:439; https://doi.org/10.1121/1.3654784.

Todd, Mabel E. (1937, Reprint 2017) *The Thinking Body*. New York, NY: Dance Horizons, Princeton Book Company.

Index

Abdomen *see also* Muscles 16, 19, 22,33–4, 44, 47, 52, 89, 101
Abdominal breathing *see* Breath
Abdominal cavity 22, 47, 52
Abdominal core 36, 39
Abdominal engagement 26, 35, 89, 97–8, 102–3, 108
Abdominal muscles *see* Muscles
Abdominal relaxation 25, 49,
Abdominal release 32, 40, 99, 102, 106
Abdominal tension 25
Abdominal viscera 44
Abdominal wall imaging 16
Alexander Technique 43
Alignment 23, 37, 43, 50–1, 56
Articulators 118
Belt 14, 19, 26, 57, 60, 85, 87, 95, 110–15
Blake, Ed. 16, 19, 23–5, 42, 46, 48-9, 61, 90
Breath
    Abdominal breathing 15, 25, 51
    Airflow 15, 17, 19, 22–5, 28–31, 35–6, 39, 44, 47–8, 59–60, 84, 86–7, 89, 94, 98, 102–3, 105, 107, 112
    Balloon analogy 15, 19, 28–9, 32, 37, 40, 46, 49, 87, 92–3
    Breathing exercise 26, 29, 31–3, 35, 38–9, 42, 47, 49, 53, 60, 87–94, 97–8
    Lungs 14, 22, 28–30, 34, 40, 44, 46–7, 49–51, 87, 92, 94, 100
    Management 103
    Subglottal pressure 17, 19, 24, 44, 46, 48, 61, 80, 95
    Resistance 16–17, 19, 24, 28–31, 34–5, 47, 59–60, 80, 84, 86–7, 89, 94, 97–8, 102–3
British Voice Association 16
Brown, Oren 42–3, 50
Bunch Dayme, Meribeth 42, 66
CCM *see* Contemporary Commercial Music
Chapman, Janice 42, 116
Constriction - *see* Laryngeal constriction
Consonant 78, 80, 97, 103, 114, 117–18
Contemporary Commercial Music (CCM) 55, 57, 89
Core stability 18, 35, 89

Cricoid cartilage 85
Dayme, Meribeth *see* Bunch Dayme, Meribeth
Deconstriction - *see* Laryngeal constriction
Diaphragm 14, 17, 19, 22, 30–1, 42–52, 60, 92–5, 99, 100
Distortion 57, 85
Dysphonia *see also* Muscle tension dysphonia 17, 61
EO *see* Muscles - External oblique
Embouchure 36, 39
Fight and flight response - *see* Performance anxiety
Finger valve breathing exercise *see* Breath - Breathing exercise
Fricative 80–1, 97, 103
'Giggle exercise' 83, 113
Glottal closure 36, 116
Hydration 61–2
IAP *see* intra-abdominal pressure
IO *see* Muscles - Internal oblique
Iliac crest 18–19, 22
Inertance 36–7, 80, 103
Intercostals *see* Muscles
Intra-abdominal pressure (IAP) 23, 52
FVF *see* Vocal folds
Laryngeal constriction 81–2, 86
Laryngeal tension *see* Muscle tension disorder
Lip trill 60, 76, 80, 86, 110
Lungs *see* Breath - Lungs
MTD *see* Muscle tension disorder
Microphone 104, 117
Morris, Ron 42, 49, 126
Muscle memory 32, 68, 96, 108
Muscle tension disorder (MTD) 23, 55–8, 61–2, 70, 82, 95
Muscles (of the abdomen) 16
    External oblique 17–18, 22, 47, 49
    Intercostals 22, 49–50
    Internal oblique 16–17, 22, 24–6, 89
    Quadratus lumborum 18
    Rectus abdominis 18, 22–3
    Serratus posterior 46

Sternocleidomastoid 24
Transverse abdominal 16–19, 22, 24–6, 31, 45–8, 52
Transversus abdominis *see* Transverse abdominal
'NG' *see* Sirening
Onset 13, 60, 77, 112–15, 117
Open vowels 59, 65–6, 68, 73, 75–6
Opera 6, 13–14, 19
PNS *see* parasympathetic nervous system
Parasympathetic nervous system 14–15, 29
Performance anxiety 14–15, 27–8, 47, 94–5, 106
Pericardium 44
Peritoneum 44
Pitch 16–17, 24, 35, 60, 69–70, 75–7, 83–4, 91, 97–8, 102–4, 108, 114–15, 117
Posture 22–3, 27–8, 43, 50–2, 120
Proprioceptor 48
Puffed cheeks exercise *see also* Breath 60, 103, 105–8
RA *see* Muscles - Rectus abdominis
Range *see* Vocal range
Register *see* Vocal register
Respiratory function *see also* Breath 12–13, 30, 32, 46, 52, 88
'Braking' 30, 49, 94
Resonance 70, 77–9, 81
SCM *see* Muscles – Sternocleidomastoid
Semi Occluded Vocal Tract exercise (SOVT) 36, 80–1, 103
Sirening 16–17, 59–60, 69–70, 73, 76–81, 84, 86, 91, 97, 110, 116
SNS *see* sympathetic nervous system
Soft palate 75–9
SOVT *see* Semi Occluded Vocal Tract exercise
Spine 19, 22, 25, 43, 46, 50, 52
Sacrum 50

Occiput 50
Steam inhalation 62, 73
Sternocleidomastoid *see* Muscles
Sympathetic nervous system 14, 28
TA *see* Muscles - Transverse abdominal
TMJ *see* Temporomandibular joint
TRT *see* Tongue root tension
Temporomandibular joint (TMJ) 66–8, 75, 110
TVF *see* Vocal folds
Thorax 22, 25, 44, 49–50
Throat valve breathing exercise *see* Breath - Breathing exercise
Thyroid cartilage 69
Todd, Mabel 43
Tongue 36, 66, 69, 75–9, 115, 117–18
Tongue root tension 13, 79, 118
Ujjayi 28, 31
Ultrasound 16, 24–5
Valsalva manoeuvre 37
Vinyasa yoga *see also* Yoga 27
Vocal folds 14–15, 27, 31, 33, 36–7, 48, 58, 61–2, 69, 80, 82–9, 95, 97–8, 103, 111–13, 116, 120
False vocal folds (FVF) 58, 82, 86, 113
True vocal folds (TVF) 82–3, 86
Vocal fry 59–60, 116
Vocal health 14, 48, 62, 78, 83, 91, 96, 119–20
Vocal hygiene 59, 61
Vocal range 3, 12, 16, 26, 35, 56–7, 69, 71, 77, 81–3, 102, 109–10, 117, 121
Vocal register 70–1, 116,
Vocal tension *see also* muscle tension dysphonia 13, 118
'VV' *see* Sirening
Yoga 1, 3, 15, 27, 45, 120
Zygomatic muscles 75
'ZZ' *see* Sirening

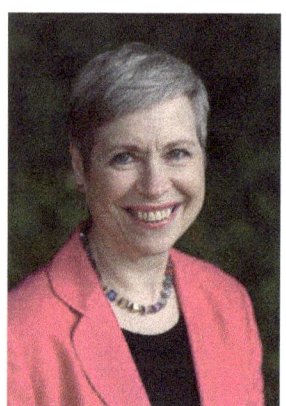

About the Author

Alison Mary Sutton, GGSM PGCA FISM, trained at the Guildhall School of Music and Drama, London, gaining honours in Graduate and Recital Diplomas and winning several major awards. As a concert singer, she has performed at most of the major London concert halls and, as part of a voice/harp duo, has fulfilled numerous recital engagements at music clubs and festivals throughout the UK. She has performed many operatic roles, working with Kent Opera, Pavilion Opera, London Opera Players, London Opera Factory and Opera de Lyon, with whom she toured in Europe and the USA. She has also sung with the Monteverdi Choir.

Alison has had a long career as a singing teacher, examiner, adjudicator, and choral workshop tutor. For many years she examined for GSM&D and for the ABRSM as a Diploma examiner. Adjudicating engagements have included Leith Hill Musical Festival and Sligo International Choral Festival. Alison ran her own residential solo singing course for several years in the Cotswolds in the UK, which was subsequently revived as part of the International Summer School of Music at Shrewsbury. She has also tutored at Hereford International Summer School and Benslow Music Trust. She was the External Specialist Assessor on the final recitals panel at Birmingham Conservatoire for several years, returning to conduct a vocal workshop, and has been on the jury for the AESS National Junior English Song Competition.

Alison is very committed to her work as the singing rehabilitation coach in the Voice Clinic at Cheltenham General Hospital and sustains a busy private rehabilitation practice.

www.ingramcontent.com/pod-product-compliance
Lightning Source LLC
Chambersburg PA
CBHW042042240426
43667CB00047B/2951